ADVANCE PRAISE FOR *THE INFLAMED FEELING*

This is a great read for those wanting a very readable insight into our inner world. Incorporating insights from psychoneuroimmunology, Mats Lekander gives us a personal tour of the way the brain experiences both our outer and inner worlds. The author includes anecdotes of his personal experiences, making the field very accessible to non-specialists as well as highly accomplished scientists.

> **Benjamin Hart**, Distinguished Professor Emeritus
> at the University of California, USA

A fascinating journey drawing together cognitive psychology, anthropology, sociology and immunology to reveal how perceptions or misperceptions of our inner world (body) impact on our health and wellbeing. A must read!

> **Neil Harrison**, Professor of Psychiatry at the Cardiff University
> Brain Research Imaging Centre (CUBRIC), UK

Join a thriller-like journey between body and brain, a constantly ongoing tourism in your innermost, in which balance and just as often unbalance is described in an accessible scientific way. Instructive and fun!

> **Barbo Osher**, philanthropist and Consul-General
> of Sweden in San Francisco

At last a book about the psychology and physiology of well-being, giving fascinating insights into questions about health which takes up so much room in contemporary society

> **Martin Ingvar**, author and Professor of Integrative
> Medicine at the Karolinska Institutet, Sweden

THE INFLAMED FEELING

the brain's role in immune defence

MATS LEKANDER

Professor of Psychoneuroimmunology, Stress Research Institute,
Department of Psychology, Stockholm University, Sweden
and
Professor of Health Psychology, Department of Clinical Neuroscience,
Karolinska Institutet, Stockholm, Sweden

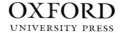

OXFORD
UNIVERSITY PRESS

Great Clarendon Street, Oxford, OX2 6DP,
United Kingdom

Oxford University Press is a department of the University of Oxford.
It furthers the University's objective of excellence in research, scholarship,
and education by publishing worldwide. Oxford is a registered trade mark of
Oxford University Press in the UK and in certain other countries

Originally published as *Ditt Inre Liv*, Mats Lekander, Fri Tanke, 2017

The moral rights of the author have been asserted

First Edition Published in 2022

Impression: 1

Published in the United States of America by Oxford University Press
198 Madison Avenue, New York, NY 10016, United States of America

British Library Cataloguing in Publication Data
Data available

Library of Congress Control Number: 2021941872

ISBN 978–0–19–886344–1

DOI: 10.1093/oso/9780198863441.001.0001

Printed in Great Britain by
Bell & Bain Ltd., Glasgow

Oxford University Press makes no representation, express or implied, that the
drug dosages in this book are correct. Readers must therefore always check
the product information and clinical procedures with the most up-to-date
published product information and data sheets provided by the manufacturers
and the most recent codes of conduct and safety regulations. The authors and
the publishers do not accept responsibility or legal liability for any errors in the
text or for the misuse or misapplication of material in this work. Except where
otherwise stated, drug dosages and recommendations are for the non-pregnant
adult who is not breast-feeding

Links to third party websites are provided by Oxford in good faith and
for information only. Oxford disclaims any responsibility for the materials
contained in any third party website referenced in this work.

PREFACE

One day during my psychology training at Uppsala University, we conducted a role play exercise in interview methodology. During the exercise, a classmate would practice interviewing a person seeking help. My role was to play a doctor with alcohol problems who had trouble acknowledging this underlying issue. During the conversation, my classmate would try to understand what I needed help with, and attempt to tease out the true problem that I struggled to articulate. But when the interview started, my partner began introducing topics that I found to be quite irrelevant. Perhaps it was his way of establishing rapport, or perhaps he thought I was concealing my true problems. He began by noting that I was a doctor. Did I also devote myself to research in my field? "Yes," I answered, a bit surprised, and thought we would move on. But instead he said, "Tell me about it." Well, I thought, I must think of something. Then it struck me that I had read, in a psychiatry textbook, that cells within the immune system can be affected by emotional processes through a kind of hormone or through neurotransmitter receptors. Complicated enough to discourage follow-up questions, I thought, as I launched into a long tirade on the subject. This should silence the inquisitive colleague. "So interesting!" the interviewer responded. But instead of moving on, he asked me to expand on the topic. I had no trouble fabricating my imaginary line of research and threw myself into the task. As I concocted a story about my exploration of emotions and immunity, I discovered that I was becoming increasingly engaged in the topic. The interviewer opened his eyes wide to the science-fiction factor of the story (and ultimately discovered my underlying problem).

I had intended to specialize in child psychology, but by the end of my training, my evolving interests had now launched me out of that track and onto a new path. This new direction was no temporary change, but became my professional self. At that time, I happened to have a father-in-law who was the Swedish government's representative in the battle against HIV. The virus was mapped, but almost nothing was known about the behavior of those who were infected or about the groups who were most at risk. The fear was great. I repeatedly came across experts who claimed that an infected person's behavior—how the patient lived his or her life—affected the progression of their illness and, more specifically, how quickly the affected person's T-cells would decrease in number until their HIV-positive status eventually turned into AIDS. A more positive attitude and robust fight against the disease was claimed to slow its development.

During our training, we were so rigorously drilled in critical thinking that we didn't believe in anything, not even in ourselves, so I was skeptical and wondered what support there was for this claim. I found, based on the newly discovered mechanisms behind how the immune system and nervous system could communicate, that it could potentially be true. But the *possibility* of being true is very different from actually *being* true, and there was in fact almost no research that showed a true connection between behavior and the development of the disease.

It resembled a popular but unproven idea at the time that cancer could be countered through grit and a positive attitude. It is understandable that doctors who work with patients observe such relationships, whether true or not. For example, you may notice cases that confirm these beliefs, or it may be that the disease affects one's behavior, rather than the other way around. I declined the offer of a paid assignment in the HIV field that would have led to a quick exam, and instead committed myself to doing something related to those small white blood cells that were alleged to be so smart. The idea of a more or less floating brain that could learn, be affected by and influence behavior, but also cause illness and suffering by misclassifying harmless stimuli as dangerous, or even cause death by missing genuine signs of danger, was spinning around in the cells in (I suppose) my own brain. But it was difficult at the time to conduct meaningful research on HIV and behavior from a *psychoneuroimmunological* (which I learned it was called) perspective, and time passed.

Instead, I began investigating the relationship between behavior and the immune system in cancer patients, and left earlier thoughts of clinical work with kids far behind. I couldn't let go of my curiosity about possible connections between the brain and phenomena in the body. Thanks to my stubborn course colleague with his surprising interview questions, those thoughts are still spinning in my head, but have taken some surprising new turns.

One of the surprises was the strong system that emanates from the body and that affects the brain and behavior. The idea that high levels of stress, emotions, or behaviors can affect our defense against disease is not new, and it is a thought surrounded by myths, hasty conclusions, and belief systems. Newer, and perhaps less surrounded by unsubstantiated claims, is the knowledge of how bodily processes such as the immune system (which is partly but not entirely located outside the brain) can control the brain. The inner world within our bodies causes us to behave in different ways—ways that over the course of development were important for our ancestors' survival. This has increased the chance for the sick to recover and for the healthy to continue to be so. The inner pressure gives rise to emotions and desires that are difficult to control—inherited tendencies that, when they function as they should, help us to survive. At the same time, the tendencies are controlled and influenced by your own experiences, by society's views about health, and by what is seen as sick or healthy at a given moment in time.

Another surprise was the discovery of systems that work proactively to maintain rather than regain good health. The study of behaviors that exist to avoid illness has quite recently gained momentum, and these behaviors are proving to have surprising consequences for attitudes toward other people, including loosely based perceptions of people who seem to deviate from our own group.

Although our conscious perception is that we have control over our behavior, it is obvious that numerous unconscious processes are at play. Some of these do not even originate in the brain but are a result of processes elsewhere in the body that preserve your health or even someone else's. This sounds undeniably strange. If true, who is "driving"? The immune system can "kidnap" the brain and cause us to behave in ways that increase our chances of recovery when we suffer from an infection. Together with norms and values that enable us to reduce the risk of becoming infected, the immune system has a surprising role in controlling our behavior, whether we want it to or not, or are aware that it is happening at all. This is reasonable from a genetic perspective, perhaps in contrast to behaviors that are supposed to preserve someone else's health, as I mentioned earlier. But the truth is that parasites—in the eternal arms race with the host animal (maybe you)—can also do their best to change your behavior. This influence from the body takes place so that the parasites can parasitize you without killing you, and in time be returned to the environment or to other unsuspecting hosts. Vomiting, sneezing, diarrhea, and so on can, in such cases, be an insidious microorganism's strategy, and thus be due to its genes and not to yours! And if we look more closely at what we in everyday speech call behavior, there are many such examples as well. Getting angry and drooling are excellent for the rabies virus, which can spread via a bite, from saliva, into the bitten animal, which thus becomes a new host where new viruses can grow. The virus affects the central nervous system of the host animal and contributes to markedly increased aggression.

Some parasites can cause an infected ant to climb high up on a leaf so that the parasites soon reach a perfect environment for reproduction—a cow's stomach! A well-known example is how the parasite *Toxoplasmosis gondii* causes rodents to stop fearing the smell of cat urine, which is perfect because the cat is the parasite's top host animal. Some studies also suggest an influence of *T. gondii* on human behavior and affection for cats. Other strange cases are wasps that can make their hosts behave like zombies and allow themselves to be guided, via their tactile rods, to the wasps' home where they then become the perfect lunch. The host animal is eaten from within in an order determined by the organs that can be eaten first without their meal (the host animal) dying. One last strikingly strange example concerns the parasite *Sacculina*, which uses parts of the female crab's reproductive system to multiply in peace while also sterilizing the crab's eggs. But if *Sacculina* ends up in a male crab instead? No problem; it simply causes a hormonal disturbance so that the crab changes sex. Personally, I think it would be easier to change host than to provoke a sex reassignment, but why not if it facilitates the transfer of genes?

Back to the immune system and its influence on what you do and feel. I'm not a zombie, you might be thinking as you read this. But you're more of a zombie than you think.

We can list examples of how phenomena in the body interact with the brain and our behavior, showing that the body's inner life is closely linked to what we want to do, to our values, and to what we choose to do. But the brain is not a passive recipient of commands from immune cells, viruses, bacteria, tumors, and other things in our inner world. It is also, to a high degree, the body's leading regulatory system, just as we have become used to seeing it. This means that the brain can start a counterattack, when appropriate, and let other motivational factors counteract the effect of an internal threat, making us behave in ways required in our daily lives—even if it hurts us and goes directly against the wishes of stakeholders within our bodies.

The subjective experience of health is central in a way that becomes clear while reading this book. If someone says that something is "only" subjective, you the reader will never again be at a loss for words. You will know why subjective health is so important and how it often overrides biological measures. The subjective experience is related in part to signals from the body, but is also dependent on the work of the brain and on factors that may have to do with society. The signals that come from the body are exposed to massive influence and control. Since this approach—our *active* interpretation of health-related signals and its biological basis—is new, I will launch a bombardment of arguments to show that I am right. What luck then that the evidence is so entertaining and thought-provoking.

During 2020 and 2021, the importance of the brain in infectious disease has been made clear across the globe. I think it is safe to say that we have focused on our bodies to detect symptoms and have tried to determine if they are signs of Covid-19 or just a consequence of poor sleep, allergy, or even increased bodily attention and expectation. We have read about, or noticed ourselves, the impact on the brain of the body's inflammatory response to the virus and the subsequent experience of malaise. Likewise, we have used behavioral avoidance to reduce the risk of becoming infected by people who may or may not carry the virus. Inflammatory responses, the brain, and behavior are intimately connected, and the relevance of this connection to your health and to your daily experiences is explained in this book.

Mats Lekander,
September 2020, Stockholm, Sweden

ACKNOWLEDGMENTS

Thanks to Lisbeth Sachs, Andreas Olsson, Martin Ingvar, Anna Andreasson, Erik Hedman, Mats J Olsson, Predrag Petrovic, and Hans Wigzell for their valuable comments. Many conversations with Arne Öhman, a true pioneer, were important in the formation of several thoughts expressed in Chapter 7. Thanks also to Emma Ulvaeus, Christer Sturmark, Rasmus Pettersson, and Lisa Swedén for their work with the Swedish edition. Thanks to Sara Aldén for copyediting my initial English translation, and Martin Baum and Rachel Goldsworthy at Oxford University Press. Thanks also to Sumathy Kumaran at Newgen Knowledgeworks as production editor, and to Carole Sunderland for copyediting.

CONTENTS

ABOUT THE AUTHOR

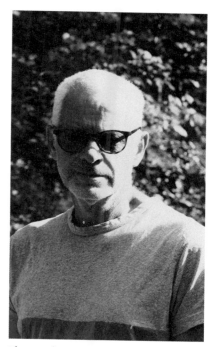

Photo: Christian Portin

Mats Lekander is Professor of Psychoneuroimmunology at Stockholm University and of Health Psychology at Karolinska Institutet Stockholm, Sweden. He is co-director of the Osher Center for Integrative Medicine at Karolinska Institutet and a former director of the Stockholm Stress Center, a center of excellence for research on work, stress, and health. He heads the Division of Psychoneuroimmunology at the Stress Research Institute at Department of Psychology, Stockholm University. His central line of research focuses on the relation between inflammation, brain function, and behavior, especially as it relates to the sickness response. He has also investigated how humans, through perceptual means, can detect when others are sick and how such detection affects behavior and attitudes. His other lines of research focus on the consequences of disturbed sleep and stress, and psychological treatment of related disorders.

LIST OF ILLUSTRATIONS

Chapter opening figures

Figures

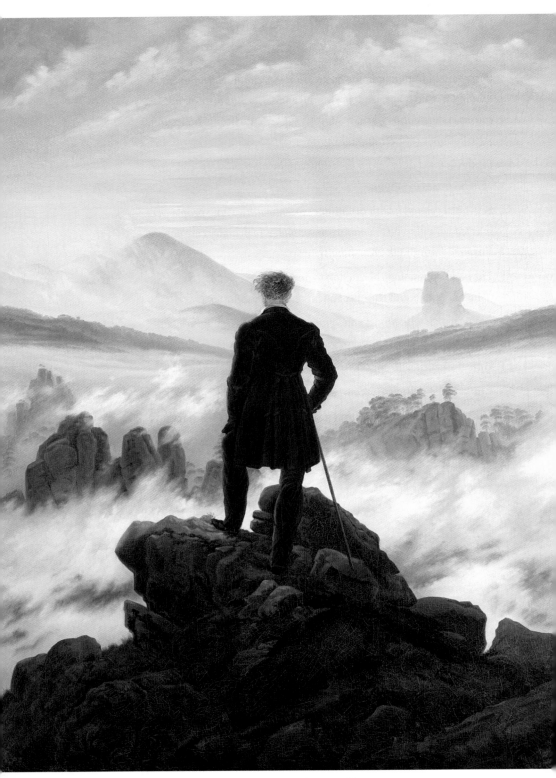

Caspar David Friedrich's "Wanderer over the sea of fog"

1

WHAT DOES THE BRAIN KNOW ABOUT THE OUTSIDE WORLD?

Observe your immediate environment for a moment—visual impressions, sounds, smells, the surface upon which you sit or stand. During this kind of exercise, you easily get the impression that you see or hear a direct reflection of reality—"das ding an sich," as the philosopher Immanuel Kant expressed in the eighteenth century. The truth, however, is that our brains construct an impression of the environment based upon information we believe is important or meaningful. Such information is selected, exaggerated, and cultivated at the expense of information that is seen as less important. The reality, as we experience it, is therefore just a guess, even if qualified and often reliable. Paradoxically, this information is not sufficient to reveal everything an individual needs to know. In spite of the enormous inflow of information, it must be complemented with guesses and assumptions in order to be useful, and adapted to our species' requirements concerning reality.

"Much information, unessential information and lack of information" are conditions under which our brains work. The fundamental nature of this guessing and construction is something that I believe I can in fact prove to you. And as luck would have it, doing so is an entertaining process. To reach my goal, I am going to use visual illustrations. But in the midst of my efforts to both entertain and inform, I hope to make an important point about how the corresponding principles also apply to the ways in which we understand our inner world. That is to say, how we understand our bodies, and therefore also our health. This phenomenon is less well known, but increasingly important in a time when we live longer,

The Inflamed Feeling. Mats Lekander, Oxford University Press. © Mats Lekander 2022.
DOI: 10.1093/oso/9780198863441.003.0001

when we can live many years with chronic disease, and when we live in a culture in which we expect a certain absence of bodily discomfort. Even though we may be missing many important pieces, we can begin to assemble a jigsaw puzzle in which a motif is clearly developing—the way in which we experience our bodies and our health, and how this experience is a construction of the brain.

The experience can be true, exaggerated, or even false. As human beings, you and I have been blessed, or perhaps cursed, with a brain that is designed to try to understand itself. This might be because we are social beings who live in pairs and in groups, who take care of helpless infants for long periods of times, and who therefore need to understand others. In order to do this, we also need to understand ourselves, in the sense that we need to read our inner states. If this leads you to think of emotions, you are on the right track. In social interactions, one must draw conclusions and make assumptions about others' inner states, needs, trustworthiness, and motives, and to a high degree we do this by simulating others' feelings and states within ourselves. The machinery needed to make assumptions about one's bodily condition is in place, and this same machinery is also used to experience, speculate, or draw conclusions about our own state of health. Thus the principles for how we do this are similar to the ones we use to understand the outer world—so let's begin there.

Interpreting the world

In psychology, the terms *bottom-up* and *top-down* are used to describe processes that deal with physical stimulations, how we experience those stimulations (bottom-up), and the processes that modulate those incoming signals and thereby the experiences themselves (top-down). A bottom-up process thus begins with the signal travelling to and entering the brain, and a top-down process with when the incoming signal is "met" by processes that emanate from the brain. Examples of top-down processes are how expectations, prior knowledge, and genetically prepared tendencies influence information that enters the brain. Top-down processes fundamentally influence how we experience the world because the information that enters the brain is often insufficient.

One example of this insufficiency is the need to see the world in three dimensions, while the projection of light onto the retina happens only in two dimensions. The projection is flat, conveying only height and width, just like onto a movie screen. Depth, however, is also needed in order to understand the shape of an object and to recognize and identify it. Depth is likewise needed for us to navigate and move about in the world. Because depth is not immediately perceived, it must be assumed and created with the help of cues and assumptions about how things should be and most often are. The fact that we have separate eyes makes it possible to produce a stereo image, which works well for shorter distances, given that the eyes are only slightly separated. The differences between the light projections that enter the left and right eyes are analyzed by nerve cells that lie next to one other in the occipital lobe in the neck. The result is one coherent image conveying depth, rather than two slightly different images. To get a sense of how much work is involved in this process, you can do a trick which challenges many assumptions.

One experiment you can do together with a friend is called the Cheshire Cat experiment (see Figure 1.1). Ask your friend to stand one or two meters in front of you against a plain surface with few distracting details—a white wall will do perfectly. While looking straight ahead at the person in front of you, position a mirror so that with the eye closest to the wall (let's say your right eye in this case) you can see only part of the wall in the mirror. With your left eye, you should see your friend's face. What will happen is that you will send completely different information (images) into a system where the information is normally the same except for a small difference in angle between each eye and the object. In addition, you will send highly interesting information for the brain (a face—perhaps the human brain's favorite object) into the left eye, and something completely uninteresting into the right. Which image will your brain choose to see? Easy, you will see the face. The "wall information" will not reach your consciousness and

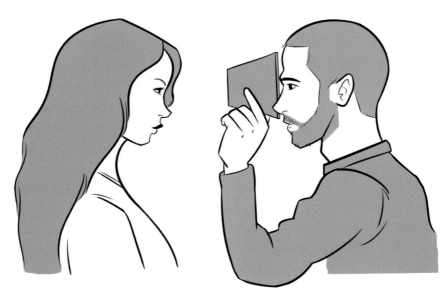

FIGURE I.I The Cheshire Cat experiment

the face will win. Now, wave your hand so that you see it in the mirror, thus sending information to your right eye. The movement attracts attention. Suddenly you will see the hand that is moving, and the neural "brake" that has stopped the information from your right eye from reaching your consciousness is gone.

Now, the fun begins. Wave a little more slowly, or ask your friend to start to talk. What do you see now? Well, it's hard to tell, but when I have done this experiment with students, we have experienced strange things when our respective brains have tried to decide what it should experience. What is coming from the left eye, the right eye, or maybe a combination of both? Perhaps a face that ends at the neck without a body, a hovering talking mouth, or a face with a waving hand instead of a nose? The phenomenon used to create this is called *binocular rivalry*—two competing images rather than two similar ones that are normally combined to create depth perception—and has been studied for many years. It shows in a dramatic fashion that the brain "constructs" an image of reality—a face or another object with a three-dimensional structure—from two similar two-dimensional images. What we see is close to the object's actual shape. With distorted or unexpected information, we can construct and experience a "reality" that does not exist, and by challenging the system we learn something about how the brain works.

We naturally strive to judge depth through the influx of information from two separate eyes into the cortex of the brain, and this tendency can be used to create three-dimensional movies so realistic that you may suddenly crouch to avoid the swarm of bees flying out of the movie screen, threatening your popcorn. The point is this: the reality we see is a calculation and no more than a smart guess.

Most cues that the brain uses to assess depth also work well at a longer distance, and are built more on logic and how something "should be" rather than real differences between the left and the right eye's respective perception of the world. My father was an engineer and familiar with stereoscopic vision, but he knew less about the multiple other depth cues that the brain can use. He was fanatically interested in tennis when Björn Borg reigned supreme, and thought it was especially impressive that Björn was so good at the sport (the world champion from 1979 to 1981, with five Wimbledon titles in a row) in spite of having such closely spaced eyes. This should have given him limited depth perception that would only work at very close distances. How could he even hit the ball?

To discuss the many cues that work well without having to use both eyes is beyond the scope of this book. But two of these cues serve as good examples because they describe phenomena that we will revisit in later chapters. One cue is about relative size and another is about position within the visual field. This means that objects that are farther away become smaller (relative to their actual size) and are projected higher up in the visual field.

If you imagine giving a speech before an audience, you probably don't believe that people in the back row are particularly small, but rather that their relative size (which is smaller) shows how far away they are compared to those (probably average-sized) individuals seated in the front rows. If we do an experiment in which distance (the depth dimension) is difficult to assess, you suddenly make important mistakes in perceiving the size of people or objects. Take a look at the illustration of a monster hunting another monster (see Figure 1.2). The monster higher up in the visual field is exactly the same size as the one farther down, but because the upper one appears to be farther away in the tunnel, and still gives a similarly large impression on the retina, it must *in reality* be much bigger than that lower one. This depth perspective is amplified by the converging lines, which contribute to the impression that the upper monster is farther away. Take a ruler and measure the size of the figures if you think this can't be true.

The monster in the upper part of Figure 1.2 thus looks bigger because it appears to be farther away. If, in spite of being farther away, it makes a similar impression on the retina, then it must be much bigger than the monster that is closer. Perhaps you are also experiencing an effect of context: which monster looks angrier, and which one looks most frightened?

The processing and construction that takes place in healthy people's brains shows large similarities and can be expressed as "laws" about how information from sensory organs should be interpreted. The modern view of perception as an active and "creative" process, building on whole objects rather than parts, and with strongly inherited features, started with the so-called gestalt psychologists in the beginning of the twentieth century. Kurt Koffka, Max Wertheimer, and Wolfgang Köhler formulated many principles for how sensory information is organized and grouped into stable shapes and patterns. One such stable unit was called a *gestalt*,[1] that is, a coherent object. These principles can, for example, be based on how similar (*law of similarity*) or close (*law of proximity*) objects are to one another, and describe tendencies to combine pieces of information into one coherent unit. Rules are needed in order to organize the messy information that reaches our brains, and, in most situations, lead us to the right conclusions with reasonable precision.

---

[1] The gestalt notion relates to the tendency to organize pieces of information into a coherent whole.

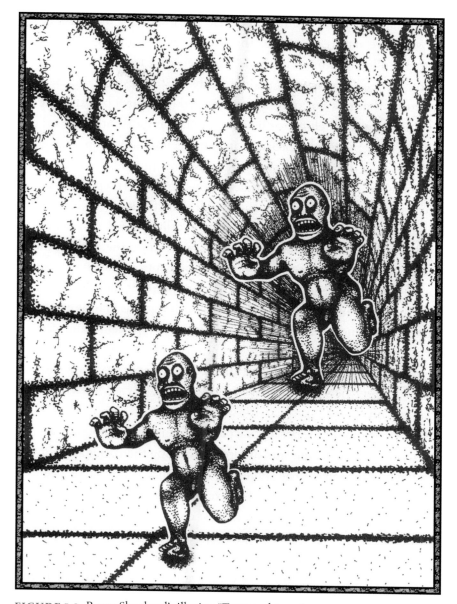

FIGURE 1.2 Roger Shephard's illusion "Terror subterra"

Shepard RN. *Mind sights: Original visual illusions, ambiguities, and other anomalies.* New York, NY: WH Freeman and Company; 1990.

Naturally, important differences also exist across individuals in the constructive nature of processing these sensory inputs—differences that are influenced by individuals' experiences, memories, and expectations at specific moments in time. Early on, the gestalt psychologists proposed that it is not only what is viewed (or heard) but also the individual who is watching (or listening) that is important. Diseases can influence the perceptual process, and changes are common after brain injuries, even though they can heal with time. Individuals with schizophrenia or autism also show deviations in the perceptual process. Because of our subjective view that we all share the same objective "impression" of reality, it is easy to believe that other people experience the world in the same way as we do. This is, however, not true, and it is therefore important to know something about perception if we are to understand the differences among people. This may be especially important if you work with unhealthy individuals where deviations may be expected. Furthermore, individual differences influence how patients' interpret information and experience bodily symptoms, such as pain or a pounding heart. Even healing processes are affected by how society, patients, and care providers view health. However, I will make a case for why this is true later on.

Knowledge about the perceptual process is important not only for understanding other people and differences among them, but also for understanding ourselves. The subjective experience is of course a central part of the perceptual process. For example, you experience the light's wavelength as a distinct quality, that is, color. You experience regular variations in sound pressure as pitch and not as variations in amplitude or vibration. On some occasions, two such aspects can be experienced simultaneously. A very low note on a grand piano—please try if you have one nearby—can be perceived both as a very low C or as a toneless flutter 16 times per second. One octave above, one would only experience pitch, and one octave below (if there were such pianos), only vibrations. The brain's perceptual process cannot make a subjectively meaningful interpretation, a gestalt, of too few cycles per second. With

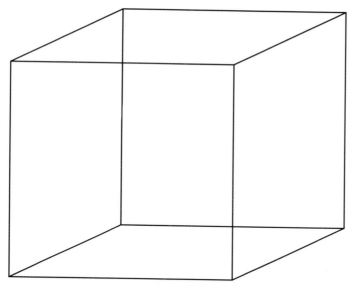

FIGURE 1.3 The Necker Cube

too many cycles per second, we can't keep track of the vibrations, and we only hear pitch.

Let me illustrate some of the simplifications and guesses that your brain performs during a typical day. The Necker cube is a well-described and widely known example (see Figure 1.3). How should you interpret this simple shape? If you study it for a while, your interpretation will change, and the corner that was closest to you will suddenly appear to be farthest away. Even though your brain will tire of the first interpretation and spontaneously change to the second,[2] you can also deliberately make the switch by focusing your attention on the corner that is farthest away. *Whoosh*—or another appropriate sound symbolizing a group of nerve cells in action—you see the cube from the other perspective. You cannot see both versions at the same time. The vagueness of the picture—that is, the lack of information guiding you toward a correct and

---

[2] For pedagogical reasons, I speak about the brain as if it was a subject of its own, rather than the "I" that is a natural aspect of the body.

stable interpretation—contributes to the instability of the gestalt, which then alternates back and forth. It is even possible to measure the activity of a group of nerve cells corresponding to one interpretation, and then compare it to that of other nerve-cell groups that are activated when your consciousness switches to the other interpretation. In this case, one can see, by studying brain activity, which interpretation you are experiencing at a given moment.

The Shephard illusion is a very powerful one, shown here (see Figure 1.4) in a simplified version in which I have included a minimum amount of cues. Look at the dimensions of the upper surface of the two boxes next to one another. How many percent longer is the long side of the left box compared to the right? The correct answer is zero—the dimensions are identical. Just as in the monster example in Figure 1.2, it is the depth that confuses your perception of reality. Because the box on the left appears to stretch away from you (and is then partly farther away), but still makes the same impression on your retina as the box on the right, it must be really long "in reality"! The length and width of the upper surfaces of the two boxes are completely identical. For those of you with inquiring minds, you can find another entertaining Shephard illusion on the internet—this one demonstrating the mistakes we can also make with our sense of hearing (though not related to depth perception).

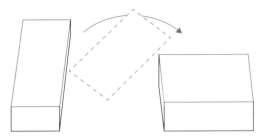

FIGURE 1.4 The Shephard illusion, inspired by Roger Shephard's "Turning the tables"

The importance of context

An important principle for how we experience the world, and which is also relevant for how you experience your body and your health, is *context*. What is the situation in which you experience something? What contextual information is available, and in what way does this context affect your interpretation? Today, we view the brain as a computational machine that not only attempts to understand the outer world (and itself, or yourself) as it truly is, but also in a way that is specific to you as an individual. What information is most important? What interpretation is safest, and what consequences did it have when you were previously exposed to this situation or object? We can, of course, view the depth information in the Shephard illusion previously mentioned as a context that guides our interpretation of size, but now we are going to take it one step further. Let's start in a simple way. Enter the Ebbinghaus illusion (see Figure 1.5).

Looking at Figure 1.5, which inner circle is largest: the one surrounded by small circles or the one surrounded by large circles? The correct answer and its interpretation are almost self-evident: namely, that the two

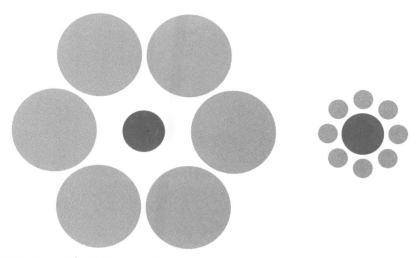

FIGURE 1.5 The Ebbinghaus illusion

inner circles are identical, and that the one surrounded by small circles is perceived to be larger because it is large in comparison to the surrounding ones. That it is *relatively* large makes us perceive it to be larger than it is, also in absolute terms. The opposite applies to the left part of Figure 1.5.

Now take a look at square A and square B in the chess board shown in Figure 1.6. Contemplate their grayness and notice the difference in lightness. In spite of the fact that they first appear to be enormously different, they are identical. If you take away the contextual information and only focus on square A or square B (for example, by observing them through a hole in a paper), it's easy to see, but the contextual information leads us astray. We are certainly of the opinion that a chess board should be lighter or darker in a well-organized grid system, but the other key factor is that the cylinder appears to cast a shadow on square B. If, in spite of being in the cylinder's shadow, it still has the light intensity that it has (the one that actually reaches your eyes), it must "in reality" be very light! Thus,

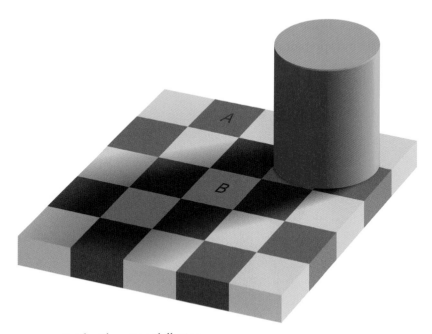

FIGURE 1.6 The Chess Board illusion

the perceptual process guides our interpretation, so that we experience square B as being much lighter than it actually is. The final result is that the exact same color is experienced as either light gray or dark gray depending on the context. This is a very clear example of the constructive nature of the work that the brain performs in order to understand the outer world and perceive it as it should be.

While it's true that visual impressions are typically consistent with reality, this is not always the case. The reason why they are so often correct is that the brain is good at guessing, compiling pieces of information, and taking effective shortcuts to make the world intelligible.

Perception without consciousness

What about subconscious processes in the brain—do they exist? The answer is yes, but unfortunately not as the exciting idea of an unconscious ego with the special task of managing intrapsychic conflicts or desires that can't bear the light of day. At least not as far as we know today.

The point is that, as a general phenomenon, the brain's processes—even those with which we perceive our own environments—are mainly unconscious. Consciousness in itself is an exception, even if it is a fascinating peephole of exception. Every moment, an enormous amount of information penetrates our brains through our sensory organs. This amount of stimulation is significantly greater than our capacity for conscious processing. While some information is prioritized and more intensely cultivated, other information is not processed at all or selected for later processing. Differences, transitions, and various types of changes are all of particular interest when trying to understand the outer world. This is because we can use this information to identify objects, people, and more out of the mess of information that reaches us through our sensory organs. There are therefore specially developed mechanisms, not only in the brain, but also in the receptors of our eyes and skin, that actively amplify differences so they are particularly apparent to us. Information that is less useful or valuable to us is suppressed. It is also possible that the information is processed outside of our consciousness. Both of these aspects appear to be true—some information is forced out because it is of limited value, and other information is processed without disrupting our consciousness. If we momentarily change perspective from the outer to the inner world, we can think about the signals the brain receives about blood pressure or oxygen levels. Isn't it good to not have to trouble our minds with every function that needs to be constantly monitored and adjusted?

If we consider something psychologically more interesting, can this take place outside of our consciousness? Yes, without any doubt. There are in fact so many examples of this that I am pausing as I write just to consider which ones to choose. Let's take something from social psychology. A group of sly students wants to test if they can control their teacher. When the teacher stands in a certain part of the classroom, the students smile more and look more interested. After a while, the teacher will have a sense that it is more rewarding to stand in that particular spot, even though she probably couldn't tell you why. Perhaps the light was better there, or it was easier to see the students from that position? Both the students and the teacher may think they know the truth, but only the students are right—the true reason is unknown to the teacher.

We can be affected by facial expressions that we do not consciously have enough time to see, or by written words that we don't have sufficient time to read and process. One technique for testing this phenomenon is called "backward masking." In this case, a stimulus is shown for a very short time, about 12 milliseconds, followed directly by a second stimulus, which is shown for a longer time and in the same part of the visual field. The result is that you only consciously see the latter stimulus, not the first. If a face with an angry expression was shown first, you can measure physiological changes demonstrating that you unconsciously responded to the threat from that face, even though you were unaware of having seen it. This technique has contributed greatly to our knowledge about neural systems, including those that control fear and anxiety.

Interestingly, it is not only when objects are shown for a very short time that visual impressions can be processed subconsciously. People with a certain type of defect in their visual system, who are blind in parts of their visual fields, are in some situations better than random at guessing what is happening in the blind spot of their visual field! This phenomenon is referred to as "blindsight"—an expression that fires up the imagination and shows how information can be accessible to us at a certain level, but still not available to our consciousness. "How could I possibly tell where in my visual field something lies if I can't see anything?" a research subject may wonder, grumbling at the stupidity of the experiment. But if she tries, she may succeed at a better-than-random rate.

A last classical example relates to how information can be accessible to us, but only in half of the brain. People with epilepsy, whose nerve connections between brain hemispheres are severed to improve disease symptoms, can sometimes perceive and know about things with one half of the brain only, if the information is presented in the part of the visual field that leads to that half of the brain. So depending on which part of the brain you "ask" (something that can be done with special techniques), you can get completely different answers! Perhaps one could say that two "consciousnesses" are then at work in the same brain?

The examples are many and most often uncontroversial, demonstrating that considerable and important aspects of how we experience our surroundings—and by extension, how we experience ourselves—take place outside of our consciousness.

The importance of expectations

Because the perceptual process is so malleable and can be affected by interpretation, context, or other factors, we can prepare the brain so that new interpretations are influenced by information that it has previously received. This type of preparation is in fact typical of the way the brain works. You can therefore influence the way the brain experiences the outer or inner world by creating expectations. For example, when we focus on an ambiguous object—perhaps a picture that can be interpreted in two different ways—we see different things in a predictable way if we first talk about or see a picture that influences our interpretation in a certain direction. Such *perceptual set* is something that can be easily influenced, and you can therefore manipulate an individual's experience. The same applies to memory functions in which you remember different things depending on your own expectations or the cues provided by another person. "Priming" is a simple way of guiding what someone will remember or attend to. The concept refers to the phenomenon that exposure to certain stimuli guides our responses to other stimuli, even though we're not aware of it. One example of this is a task in which you are asked to fill in two missing letters between "b" and "k" in order to spell a word. If you first saw a list of words related to reading, you would probably think of the word "book," but if you were encouraged to think about money, chances are you would instead complete the word as "bank." Priming is sometimes used by magicians so that they can predict responses or choices by an audience member and make it appear as though they are reading minds. One effective way to create expectations is through associations, known as conditioning, which—just like priming—can take place consciously or subconsciously.

Because expectation is such a basic human principle, it is natural that it is involved in both how we experience our surroundings and how we experience ourselves and our bodies. We will return to this subject in due course.

The dominance of the visual system

What happens if a certain sensory system receives information that collides with information we receive via another perceptual system? On such occasions, the brain must decide which information should represent reality. If you watch a ventriloquist, you will experience that spoken sound comes directly from the mouth of the doll and not from the ventriloquist, because you will observe the mouth of the doll moving in a way that corresponds to the pattern of the sound. This sound seems, so to speak, directed from the doll to your ears. In a similar way, you will experience the voice of a singer as coming directly from the performer, not from the loudspeakers on the edge of the stage or the ceiling, which in reality transmit nearly all the sound that reaches your ears. These examples remind us of when the right and left eyes receive contradictory information (as in the Cheshire Cat example; see Figure 1.1)—the brain must choose a reasonable representation of reality. The ventriloquist and the singer also demonstrate how the visual system can dominate and take precedence over other systems. Information from the visual system can also be used to make a person experience their body differently, as I will describe in the next chapter.

Thus . . .

Classic perceptual psychology clearly shows how the brain actively forms opinions about the world based on estimations, and in making these estimates, information that is judged to be the most reasonable is used. Top-down processes, as they are called, are fundamental to human perception. Once you begin to dive more deeply into these questions, you may ask yourself if this principle only applies to the way in which you experience your environment, or if the same principle might also apply to how you experience yourself, and even your personal health.

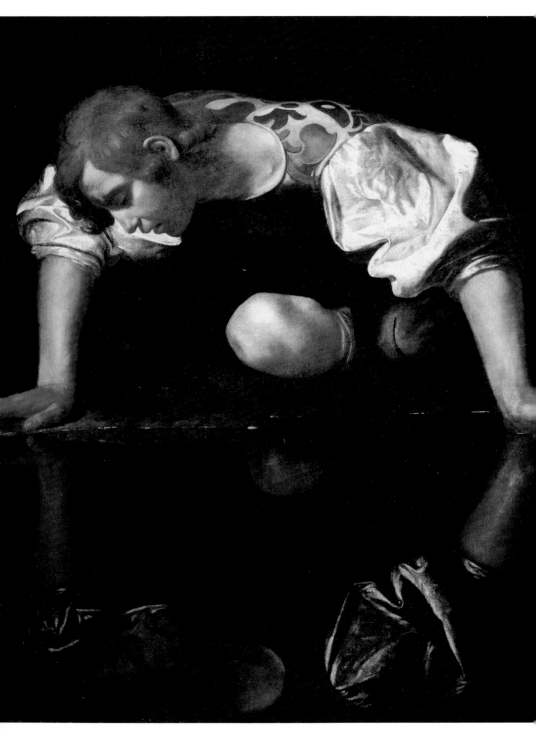

Michelangelo's Merisi da Caravaggio's "Narcissus"

2

WHAT DOES THE BRAIN KNOW ABOUT THE BODY?

I remember one afternoon during my college years when, like so many other days, I was in a hurry to catch the train after the day's lectures. I could catch an early train if I ran to the station, almost breathless, with my favorite red book bag flapping on my shoulder. Uneasiness spread throughout my body, but if I could catch the earlier train, I wouldn't have to wait an extra hour at the station. Why was everything so uncomfortable, in spite of the fact that I was just running? Why was I filled with such a negative feeling? The same activity, minus the book bag on my shoulder, would feel utterly different if I were merely out for a jog. I preferred other forms of exercise to jogging, but even that was pure pleasure as compared to the experience of racing against the clock to catch a train while contemplating if it was futile or not. Instead, I imagined that I was not in fact running for the train, but in the woods or in another scenic place. As if by a stroke of magic, the whole experience transformed, and the physical sensation was no longer stress, but exercise. All unpleasantness disappeared, and I repeated the trick every time thereafter that I hurried to the station. The whole phenomenon is a good example of a top-down process where one uses a strategy that allows the brain to receive and reinterpret the body's signals (tiredness, pounding heart, perhaps minor pain) in a new way. A so-called higher brain function governs and reinterprets these signals. Perhaps the principles needed to understand the outer world that I described in Chapter 1 also apply to

The Inflamed Feeling. Mats Lekander, Oxford University Press. © Mats Lekander 2022.
DOI: 10.1093/oso/9780198863441.003.0002

information coming from the body? Moreover, perhaps this also applies to how we view our health.

Interpreting the body

On one level, my experience of running at full speed from Uppsala University's Department of Psychology to the city's train station is a trivial observation, even though dramatic in the everyday life through which my body navigated. The academic literature on stress refers to this known phenomenon as *appraisal*. The *individual person* who is exposed to a stressor, and their unique interpretation of that event, among other factors, influences the stress response. Perceived control affects the response—that is, one's belief in being able to influence a stressful situation or not. How big is the threat in light of my perceived power to influence it? How predisposed am I to anxiety? How do I interpret the stressor in relation to my resources, and what do I think will be the outcome? These types of individual factors influence the amount of stress hormones that will be released, or how much the autonomous nervous system and the immune system will be activated. In addition, they play a clear role in the experience itself. Now we're approaching the heart of the matter. With the concept of appraisal, one's subjective experience, conscious or not, becomes integrated with the definition of stress. The process is an example of an emotional coping strategy[1] in which the emotional response—but neither behavior nor the stress-inducing event—is changed.

On another level, the example tells us much about our attitude toward our bodies. We filter signals that come from within our bodies in the same way as we filter those that come from the external world—the same sort of journey that signals from the outer world experience as they travel

---

[1] *Emotional coping* refers to a way of dealing with an upsetting or uncomfortable situation by managing the emotions that the situation provokes. To paraphrase stress researcher Lennart Levi, if one decides to change the shoe that doesn't fit rather than reshaping one's foot, you are using *problem-focused coping*. If I had decided to leave earlier for the train, that would be an example of the latter strategy, not a top-down process in its usual sense.

from receptor (perhaps a cone or rod in the retina of the eye) to interpretation (within and between different brain areas) and over to experience. Compare this to the Gestalt psychologists' view that it is not only the object itself but also the person that influences the end result when it comes to comprehending the outer world.

Okay, so send signals from the outer world into the system, get rid of the ones that seem unimportant, focus on changes and transitions, prepare the body for what is coming, and pay attention to things that build on what you think you know or expect will happen. You don't see with your eyes, but with your brain. This means that the stream of signals from the outside is met by other internal signals and is modified during its journey toward our consciousness, or for that matter, toward the stimulation of a behavioral response. The end result is not a direct response to an objective reality, but is a practical and often successful approach to dealing effectively with the environment.

The downside? Well, take your pick. The consequence of the tendency to confirm existing beliefs is that one becomes more easily prejudiced. For example, because you tend to focus on things that confirm your beliefs, you see and experience individual and facial features less effectively in a person from an ethnic group other than the one you grew up with, and it's more difficult to extinguish fear that you may associate with this person. Another downside is the tendency toward fallacies. An example is a witness to a traffic accident who you believe will testify on your behalf during the police inquiry, but who experiences and remembers things differently than you do depending on their preconceived notions about you—quite interesting and effective examples of the consequences of having a brain that is predisposed to shortcuts (but in essence another story).

An important question is if such top-down phenomena may also apply to the inner world—your own body. If you consider the vast, albeit incomplete, flow of information to the brain, the process cannot differ greatly when we're talking about the inner environment. Psychology and neuroscience have been late in applying the same systematic perspectives used to understand the processing of information from the outer world to the inner world.

By combining older and newer academic and empirical psychology with methods for studying how the brain works, we can achieve small wonders. In fact, science is now in a position in which subtle phenomena can be studied without having to dedicate oneself to religious or meta-physical ideas. But "the harder the subject, the more rigorous the methods that are needed," as a colleague of mine often says. If the subject is diffi-cult, it shouldn't be handled with sloppy methods, guesswork, or beliefs in things that are colored by our values. On the contrary, it should make us even more scrupulous.

On innumerable occasions, I have been in meetings with skilled scientists who have suddenly abandoned their scientific standards when the subject has become difficult yet familiar—as in the case of psychology—instead of the other way around.

The brain's attempts to understand the body

The sensation of stimuli coming from inside the body is called *interoception*. It corresponds to the word "perception," which relates to sensations coming from the outer world. Sometimes the word *exteroception* is used in-stead of perception to underscore its relationship to information coming from the outside, just as interoception refers to information coming from within the body. Originally, interoception denoted information from the *viscera*, that is, the inner organs, such as the heart or the lungs in the chest, and the intestines in the belly. But something has happened to the concept, reflecting new knowledge about how we experience our bodies. The con-cept of interoception has widened to now also denote the perception and integration of information from the whole body. For phenomena that are related to the outside of the body, there is a clear mapping of exactly where on the body something is happening, for example on the skin. Every part of the body has a clear corresponding area on the cortex, and it is well known that some areas, like the face and fingers, are represented by bigger cortical areas than others, and therefore have a higher resolution. But the inside of the body is not as clearly mapped, and the localization of, for example, pain in an inner organ—exactly where it hurts—is less distinct from a spatial perspective. Arguably, you can do less with the information of where it hurts when it is inside the body, so natural selection has apparently not favored high-resolution mapping of inner parts of the body. We can see this in the brain's organization, and it is logical that we keep track of where *on* the body something is happening (perhaps you want to direct motor activity to quickly get rid of an insect) as compared to events felt within the body that are out of reach. At the same time, systems conveying messages from within the body exist to influence our behavior in other ways, through what we sense and how we feel. A range of important signals from the body are there to inform the brain about its condition. The brain's major task, it is sometimes argued, is to keep the body's physiological systems in balance and to interpret and to respond to them in an effective manner. The signals that the brain receives are often quite diffuse, and one can reasonably argue that top-down processes take on an even more important role when trying to interpret diffuse signals, allowing the brain more leeway for interpretation.

As humans, we are equipped with a distinct neural system to send information from the body to the brain and for the subjective experience of bodily state. Interestingly, some areas that receive information about the inner world (interoception) are adjacent to areas that interpret the outer world (exteroception). An area that plays a central role in interoception is the insular cortex. It is folded within the cortex and cannot be seen from outside of the brain without separating the parietal cortex and the temporal cortex. The insula is activated by a range of phenomena that involve subjective judgment as well as experiences involving the body and emotions (which also involve the body). Pain, breathlessness, heat, cold, nausea, hunger, thirst, sexual arousal, anger, taste (and the related emotion of disgust), judgment about others' feelings, and so on, all involve the insular cortex.

The insula is a large area of the brain, and there is one in each hemisphere. Not surprisingly, the different parts of the insular cortex serve different functions. The division of labor appears to be that the posterior (rear) part primarily receives information "as it is," and the anterior (front) part processes information and puts it in a larger context. The posterior (rear) part thus works in a way that is more bottom-up, while the anterior (front) part is more top-down.

Here, the organizational principle and division of labor also remind us of how the brain tries to understand the outer world. The organizational model describing how the brain perceives the outer world (exteroception) has been well known and documented for many years. After being received by receptor cells in sensory organs and processed through relay stations such as the thalamus, the information reaches a first and so-called "primary" area in the cortex. For the visual system, this area resides in the occipital lobe. After reaching the primary cortical area, information is forwarded to other areas. The different areas work together to create a useful representation of the world, and influence one another at the same time. In the beginning, the information is not well processed, but as the information continues along the path and reaches the frontal areas of the brain, the abstract picture becomes increasingly clear. The *significance* that viewers assign to what they see, together with their understanding of it, play an increasingly important role. For example, the specific object or person you look at, and what it means to you, are now processed and coded. Typically, this analytical process progresses when the information moves forward through the brain.

Another aspect is that emotions and memories are increasingly important in the process. One example that relates to Chapter 1 is about the way in which we perceive distance. When we see an object, the neurons in the retina and primary visual cortex are activated. The extent of the activation corresponds directly to the amount of light that enters the eye from the object itself. Therefore an object that is far away activates a smaller area than if it were closer to you. With this type of information, we can build up an image of the world and eventually identify the object. But what if the object in question is your best friend? You should perceive your friend in the same way, and to be the same size, regardless of how close or far away she or he is. Thus, distance, light conditions, and similar factors are "removed," and you perceive the person in the same way regardless of the temporary variations of the information that reach your eye. The further in the processing, the less the circumstances matter, and the more what the object is believed to be like in "reality." Many of the illusions in Chapter 1 relate to what happens when this process of abstraction—our attempt to make sense of the world—fails and the system is strained.

A system similar to the one used for exteroception also plays an important role in interoception. The rear part of the insula can be seen as a primary cortical area, but in this case for information from within the body rather than from the outer world. Information is processed in an increasingly complex way within a network of areas, just as it is in exteroceptive processes. One of these areas with a complex job description is the front part of the insula. Subjective experiences related to the body usually involve the anterior insula. Together with other parts of the network, a sense of the body's physical condition is developed and—importantly—an assessment made of if behavior needs to be adjusted. Should one's bodily experience have any consequences? Should one adjust behavior so that the same phenomenon can be avoided in the future? An important aspect is whether the bodily condition one experiences differs from what was expected. A sense of surprise, in that case, might lead to some kind of behavioral change, or to an updated inner model of the world, so that expectations are more correct the next time. What behavior could be changed? One might avoid the same action as before, repeat a behavior that felt good, or do something about the physical symptoms experienced that were interpreted as symptoms of sickness or decay.

When interoceptive stimuli are processed in the insula, it is, as noted, executed in collaboration with other areas of the brain. In short, interaction with the cingulate cortex is believed to be related to motivation and to choosing a behavioral response to the information coming from the body. For example, you could do something that stops a sensation of pain. It is thought that interaction with the orbitofrontal cortex deals with evaluation in terms of good or bad (reward and punishment) and expectations. How does my experience of my bodily state match my expectations, and is my experience compatible with my goals? The anterior cingulate and the orbitofrontal cortex influence the activity in the anterior insula, the evaluation of one's bodily condition, and the consequences of this assessment.

The dramatic importance of one's subjective interpretation of physical sensations recently became even clearer to me. One day at work, I suddenly noticed how my body seemed to protest when I moved. My stiff painful muscles and joints seemed to resist all movements. Suddenly, I became aware of a growing discomfort that had been there for some time, but that I had not really noticed until then. I thought to myself, now I am deteriorating. I have passed the better part of middle age. The lasting stiffness will only get worse, and what I now expect is nothing less than going to the dogs. Depressing thoughts, no doubt. I concluded that it was all downhill from there, and it had never been as obvious as it was just then. But after a while, I started to consider what I had done the day before. Hadn't I biked manically to the tennis courts, duelled with a much younger friend for over three hours, and then biked back all the way through Stockholm (one of the world's least flat capitals)? Great, I thought, maybe things are looking up again. The physical message I received, as seen through my humble middle-aged office perspective, was this: I am getting even stronger! I stretched and raised my head a little higher—in the end, a pretty good day at work!

A simplified interpretation of that experience in "neuro-lingo," based on our understanding today, would look something like this: The pain and stiffness signals are sent to the posterior and middle parts of the insula. The anterior parts of the insula are responsible for an important part of the subjective experience and for the astonishment at the bodily discomfort (*ouch—I'm so stiff, should it be like this?*). The anterior insula, together with the cingulum, interprets the behavioral relevance—what action the sensation should lead to. (I am deteriorating and soon done. What should I do? Eat differently, google "rheumatism," or just lie down and give up?) Together with the orbitofrontal cortex, an interpretation is then made to decide if it is good or bad (bad!) and if it is in line with my expectations of how I believe I should feel—that is, my goal was to be more mobile, but maybe it's unrealistic to expect that in this phase of life? When the context changes (when I remember yesterday's efforts), the signals are reinterpreted as ordinary exercise pain and as a sign that things are in fact improving. At that moment, the "danger value" of the bodily signals ceases. I do not need to change my behavior and can think of something else. That interpretation takes place in the outer parts of the orbitofrontal cortex and in the anterior cingulum, and affects the activity of the anterior insula. The discomfort is suddenly experienced almost as a reward. I no longer need to think about the signals from my body, whose tireless shouts of "Hello! Pay attention!" gradually taper off. I can continue with what I was doing before, reassured that everything is back to normal, if not better.

My interpretation and control over a physical experience is obvious when I run to catch a train and when I try to understand the cause of my wayward body. In the train example, I did an active and deliberate reinterpretation, and in the tennis example, I refined my explanatory model. As a result of top-down processes, my perception of my body's condition changed significantly.

Research on regulation and control of emotions has understandably become very active. Some regulation happens more automatically, for example when emotionally interesting stimuli (which easily attracts our attention) need to be ignored in order to not interfere with another function, such as an assessment. Another type of regulation is about cognitive reappraisal, which was what I was doing when I pretended that I was running in the woods instead of racing for the train. When I perform a cognitive reinterpretation (reappraisal), it is a more conscious and proactive process, where I change the rules for how something should be interpreted. If we measure this process with functional magnetic resonance imaging, the subject can imagine that a distraught man in a photo is actually crying with happiness, or that a burning house is part of a movie set instead being someone's home. This leads to a weaker emotional response.

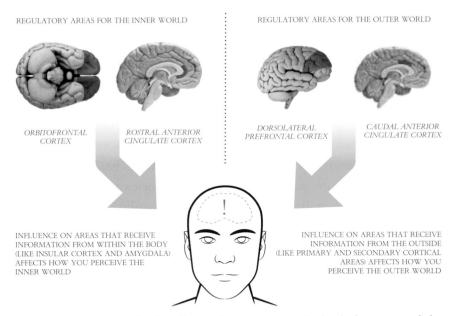

REGULATORY AREAS FOR THE INNER WORLD

REGULATORY AREAS FOR THE OUTER WORLD

ORBITOFRONTAL CORTEX

ROSTRAL ANTERIOR CINGULATE CORTEX

DORSOLATERAL PREFRONTAL CORTEX

CAUDAL ANTERIOR CINGULATE CORTEX

INFLUENCE ON AREAS THAT RECEIVE INFORMATION FROM WITHIN THE BODY (LIKE INSULAR CORTEX AND AMYGDALA) AFFECTS HOW YOU PERCEIVE THE INNER WORLD

INFLUENCE ON AREAS THAT RECEIVE INFORMATION FROM THE OUTSIDE (LIKE PRIMARY AND SECONDARY CORTICAL AREAS) AFFECTS HOW YOU PERCEIVE THE OUTER WORLD

FIGURE 2.1 Circuits that handle top-down processes for both the outer and the inner world.

Inspired by Predrag Petrovic, adaptation by Rasmus Pettersson. Images: Shutterstock

In such studies, it is possible to see that certain parts of the frontal lobes, such as the orbitofrontal cortex, are important to this interpretation. My orbitofrontal cortices did an excellent job during my run, as my re-interpretation dramatically changed the experience. Other parts of the frontal lobes, such as the anterior cingulum, are also involved in regulating both emotional and other bodily processes, such as pain (Figure 2.1). We will return later to the theme of emotional regulation, in part to understand how we perceive the body when we are sick, and partly to see how psychological treatment can help people by affecting their interpretation of the inner world.

The mapping of mechanisms at play in the inner world (see left part of Figure 2.1) has also begun. Here too, the signal (such as a pain signal in the spinal cord) can be up- or downregulated even before it reaches the brain. "Higher" brain areas such as the orbitofrontal cortex and rostral anterior cingulum (see Figure 2.2) can control other areas, such as the

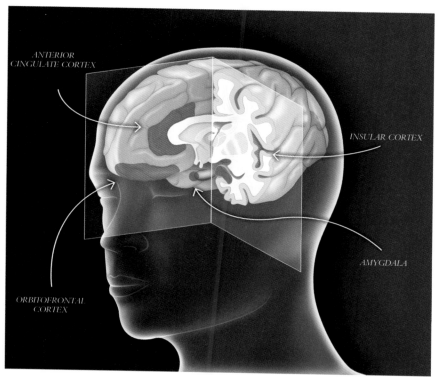

FIGURE 2.2 Model of the brain, with the front part of the left hemisphere removed to show more clearly where some relevant parts are located. In the frontal part of the brain, the orbitofrontal cortex and cingulum are visible; inside the temporal lobe, the amygdala can be seen. Between the parietal and the temporal lobes, the insula can be glimpsed, which also continues forward between the frontal cortex and the temporal lobe.

Mats Lekander and Rasmus Pettersson. Image: Sciencephoto

insula (see Figure 2.3) or amygdala, or areas of the brain stem. Attention, which is controlled in these and other areas of the brain, greatly affects what signals are perceived, and how strongly, regardless of where they originate.

I wrote that the insula is a fairly large cortical area. In fact, it is greatly magnified in humans in relation to what one could expect when compared to the brains of other primates. It may have to do with the fact that we are social beings who need to understand both ourselves and each other in order to function in groups. Similarly, people's respective insula areas differ

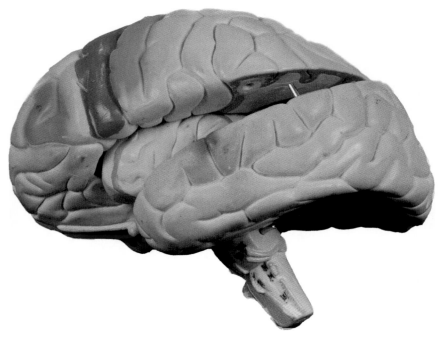

FIGURE 2.3 The insula is a part of the cortex but is not visible from outside of the brain. When I have opened my model of the brain along the side, the insula becomes more clearly visible.

Photo: Tina Sundelin

greatly in how they are structured—they simply look different. It is tempting to conclude that this corresponds to differences in how they function in different people and to how sensitive we are to bodily information. Individual variation could be related to its size and structure, and to the variable form of other parts of the cortex. Some evidence supports this conclusion. Brains are as different from one another as faces, it is sometimes said, and it is clear if you look at pictures of different individuals' insular areas.

Does the body exist?

Experiencing a body part that does not exist, and feeling pain or itching in that area, is a troublesome and dramatic reminder that our brain's perception of the body is not one hundred percent accurate. Small variations on this theme can be experienced by everyone, such as when you have been lying or sitting very quietly and feel that a body part has a different size than normal, or that its perceived location does not correspond to reality. For example, you may be resting in bed and suddenly feel like your body is a little twisted, though it is not. Such experiences are not uncommon when you are falling asleep, and the absence of movement gives your brain fewer clues to construct a reasonable picture of the position of your limbs or the shape and size of your body. A more dramatic experience has been reported by people who are about to undergo arm surgery and whose sensation is knocked out with a nerve block. The patient raises their arm when the block is administered. When they lower their numb arm, they often remark, "Strange, it feels like . . . " the healthcare provider easily finishes their sentence: "...like you're still holding up your arm?" The patient looks surprised and asks how the person could know. But the phenomenon is quite common. The memory of the arm's position prior to the nerve block remains and is not replaced by new information after the arm is numbed and lowered. The "old" knowledge of the arm's position is the brain's best available information and "wins" over the visual information of the arm's new position. In the absence of updated information, the brain creates a model of the body that does not correspond to reality. What else would it do? Not provide any opinion at all due to a lack of reliable data? Hardly.

Similar phenomena occur after amputations, where the absence of information from the real body part causes memories and beliefs—or perhaps random phenomena—that make us think, for example, that a removed hand is tightly knotted in a fist. Phantom experiences are not uncommon after amputations, and pain in body parts that no longer exist is a clinical problem. However troublesome they may be for the afflicted person, phantom phenomena are philosophically interesting. A classic thought experiment on a "phantom body" is to think about what happens if you first amputate a finger, then a hand, then an arm, and then further parts of the body. How much of the body can be a phantom experience?

In some ways, it is not surprising that one can experience body parts that do not exist. The perception of the body must be changeable because we grow, train, develop bigger muscles, or perhaps become injured. Therefore we must have a malleable, that is, changeable, representation of our body parts in the brain. If we practice a task, such as trying to recognize shapes using our fingers instead of our vision, or distinguishing different musical pitches, the size of the brain areas that receive information from the fingers changes. Areas of the brain that are normally less involved in these activities may even be drawn into the surrounding areas' tasks. The task being trained seems to need increased process power and to dispose of larger amounts of the cerebral cortex than those not being trained. These processes can, to a limited extent, occur quite quickly, but we may also see large and long-lasting changes, especially if we start training early in life. A well-researched example concerns the effect of musical training. If we study the fingers' sensory representation in the brain of a string musician, we can see that the fingers used to press down the strings on the finger-board clearly have greater representation areas compared to the thumb on that hand (which is typically used as support on the neck of the finger-board), or compared to the corresponding fingers on the other hand. The earlier you start playing as a child, the greater the effect. In addition, the sooner you start playing, the greater the probability of developing per-fect pitch.

So, what does it mean for us that we may feel sensations from hypothetic fingers, and experience an itch or pain in non-existent body parts? If an area of the brain no longer receives information from the body part in question, the area can be taken over by surrounding brain areas that re-ceive information from other parts of the body. It is thought then that the experience does not have to accompany the new source of the signal. The activity in the area is interpreted as "as usual," that is, as if it originated from the amputated body part. Simply put, you now have activity in a part of the brain that normally comes from a specific body part. The signal comes from another body part that has now partially "invaded" the representa-tion area in the cerebral cortex. The result is that you find that something is happening in the body part that no longer exists. It is possible to provoke a sensation in an amputated hand by poking part of the face with a wet cotton swab. Inside the brain, the face is represented next to the hand, and it may be that one experiences something wet not only on the face but also in the hand that no longer exists.[2]

Thus the body experience is not a direct reflection of the physical reality, but a calculation. The body is a hypothesis—once again, one that is normally reasonable and well-functioning, but sometimes completely inaccurate, with a potential for both ill health and recovery that is of great relevance to medical practice.

One way to change this calculation following an amputation is through mirror therapy. If a patient perceives that their amputated hand, let's say the left one, is cramped and contorted, a mirror can be placed vertically between the hands, facing the right hand. The right hand is then clenched in the same way as the phantom hand, looking in the mirror as though the left hand were still in place. When the patient slowly opens his hand, it looks as though the missing hand is now moving. In successful cases, the sensation of the cramped hand gives way, the movement of the phantom hand appears to return, and the pain can disappear. The visual impression of movement helps the brain interpret the sensation from the body: the mirrored right hand must in fact be your actual left hand. The method is not fully tested and confirmed, but serves as an example of a top-down process related to body perception—one that brings us a step closer to understanding how our "inner" world is created, and what role interpretations and beliefs play in these processes.

---

[2] Some obscene examples corresponding to how we think this works have been provided by the scientist and maverick Vilayanur S. Ramachandran, who Richard Dawkins called "the Marco Polo of neuroscience": Some people with lower leg amputations reported, in letters to Ramachandran, that the experience of an orgasm was no longer limited to the genitals but in fact also experienced in the phantom foot. A probable explanation is that the foot is represented next to the genitals in the somatosensory cortex of the brain, so that stimulation from the genitals also causes activity in the area originally devoted to the foot.

(Ramachandran VS, Blakeslee S. Phantoms in the brain: Probing the mysteries of the human mind. New York: William Morrow, 1998.)

Where is the body, whose is it, and which one is mine?

So, if the body is a hypothesis, then we should be able to push the system to make interesting mistakes. Through controlled experiments, we can induce the kinds of bodily illusions that have been carried out for many years to understand how our senses of vision and hearing are structured. At Henrik Ehrsson's lab at Karolinska Institutet in Stockholm, a large number of experiments such as these have already been carried out. Perhaps best known is the rubber hand illusion, which his research group has further developed through several experiments. During these experiments, the subject sees a rubber hand in front of them on a table, while the individual's own hand is hidden by a screen. In place of their own hand, a mock hand can thus be seen. If the rubber hand is touched synchronously—that is, in pace with the real hand—the person's sense of sight will soon override their sense of touch in determining the origin of the sensation. They feel the touch in their real hand, which is hidden, and see the rubber hand touched at the same moment as the real hand. Abracadabra, you gain "ownership" of the rubber hand—together with a sense of touch through that hand—rather than through your real hand. During this illusion, you may also experience strong autonomous reactions if, for example, your precious rubber hand is threatened with a blow from a hammer. Thus, sight can control and reorganize sensory impressions from an individual body part and influence the experience.

But the sense of ownership of the *whole* body can also be transferred to someone else's body, or even to a pretend body. In another experiment, the subject puts on virtual-reality glasses that are connected to a video camera, so that they see exactly what the camera sees. The camera can then be placed so that it "looks down on" the upper body and legs of a mannequin, as if you were looking down over your own body. The pretend body may be a different size than the actual one, it still works. Even a small Barbie doll can be successfully used in this body ownership illusion—an identity-based quantum leap that the brain can perform just like that. In Chapter 1, I wrote about how eyesight can control other senses, such as hearing. The examples in this chapter clearly show that you can redefine your own body, and even adjust the experience so that it matches the visual impression.

When we can experience dead objects as if they were body parts, or transfer a whole-body experience to a small doll, one can conclude that the experience of the body, like other parts of the world, is an active calculation. We use the information we have and make the most of it. Sensations in the body give us a lot of important clues about how we should behave, and how we should interact with other people and with the outside world. How steep is the hill we see in front of us? The hill actually looks steeper if we put on a heavy backpack. The assessment depends not only on our visual impression, but also on the physical assessment of how difficult it would be to climb.

The placebo effect

The concept of placebo refers to a positive consequence of a treatment that does not result from the treatment itself. The treatment is, in some cases, a drug, but can in fact be virtually any treatment. The term "nocebo" stands for negative effects that are not caused by the treatment, but is basically the same as placebo. The term is said to have been associated with behaviors related to cheating and simulation after hired mourners in the thirteenth century chanted a psalm verse that began "Placebo Domino" (I will please the Lord).

Placebo effects can be repeatedly demonstrated in well-controlled experiments, and several mechanisms underlying the phenomenon can be understood. One can also knock out the effects pharmacologically by blocking the receptors involved in a particular mechanism. The effects in the brain can be measured, or studied at a subjective level, so it is clear that the placebo effect is "real." In everyday life, you may also feel stimulated by decaffeinated coffee, or perhaps feel the effects of caffeine through the smell alone as you bring the cup to your mouth.

Placebo effects are brilliant examples of how top-down processes modify signals coming from the body and how these signals are subjectively perceived. The change is of course physiological—it is created by chemical and electrical changes in different parts of the body, even when we can only observe the effect subjectively through our own personal experience. The whole phenomenon fits well with the general modus operandi of the brain including shortcuts, expectations, preparation, overarching control, and learned automated responses.

The top-down effects that are at the heart of placebo are usually seen as driven by two main mechanisms. The first is expectation, like when you believe that a certain drug should work because you know that it is usually prescribed for a particular health problem. The second mechanism is conditioning—the associative learning that Pavlov explored with his dog experiments. Both expectation and conditioning are parts of the brain's general tendency to try to predict events and react to them well in advance. To achieve this general aim, several mechanisms are used. In many cases, the brain and other parts of the body begin reacting physiologically to events before they have actually occurred. There is more than one way for the brain to control the body and to simulate an event without it actually occurring. The most basic associative learning mechanisms even work nicely on very simple organisms with no traditional brains and few nerve cells.

A classic way to trigger a placebo effect is to administer saline or an inert pill to a person who thinks they are receiving a proper medication. A Swedish study by Predrag Petrovic and colleagues on pain relief through placebo showed that roughly the same area of the brain, the anterior cingulum, was successfully activated by a placebo as when a morphine preparate was given. This area of the brain has previously been activated for pain relief through hypnosis or distraction, and is known to be part of the brain's pain inhibition system. Together with other studies, the Swedish study demonstrates that a control station for pain can be activated by either placebo or medication; in either case, it can lead to pain relief. In this example, it is a conscious expectation (about pain relief) that triggers a top-down mechanism that reduces the pain experience. But then a question arises: can placebo effects be triggered more automatically and perhaps completely unconsciously? The answer is yes, and aspects of the body's healing processes in the immune system have been shown to be amenable to modification in such ways.

It is amazing how much knowledge of the nervous system and behavior emerged after the innovative and hugely productive Ivan Pavlov described how his dogs learned to initiate a variety of physiological reactions in response to environmental signals. If the dogs learned that the sound of a bell was a reliable signal for receiving food, they prepared for digestion and began salivating after hearing the sound but before any food appeared. After his Nobel Prize in Physiology for discoveries about digestion, Pavlov produced several hundred articles on learning—that is, the form of learning that was subsequently called Pavlovian, or classical, conditioning. Thanks to the rigorous methods Pavlov developed (and indirectly to his abandonment of earlier studies on both digestion and theology), discoveries about learning, memory, and the brain's fear system have taken huge strides forward. The term "Pavlov's dog" is now well established in popular culture.

Less well known is that Russian researchers such as Makukhin, Metalnikov, and Chorine, who succeeded Pavlov, studied whether the immune system could also be influenced through conditioning, and whether the production of antibodies was a conditioned reflex. Antibodies can be described as receptors that can neutralize a microbe or tag it for other parts of the immune system. It was argued that perhaps these antibodies were influenced by learning and by the nervous system. Despite some positive early results, the idea of immune system conditioning did not fit neatly with the dominant ideas of the day about immune system processes, and was discarded. In the field of immunology, the white blood cells were primarily studied in test tubes and not in the physical environment in which they actually exist—inside bodies such as mine and yours.

An environment where hormones, nerves, and thereby behaviors that intersect may be part of the equation.

Ideas related to the brain's regulation of the immune system (and vice versa) did not take off until the 1970s, due in part to American psychologist Robert Ader's argument that some phenomena observed in his animal experiments could be explained by immune system conditioning, reasonably then involving the brain. The rats had been given a sugar solution just before they received a substance that made them nauseous. This was done to study how taste can cause avoidance, even if the taste is followed by nausea not until several hours later. The phenomenon is called taste aversion and is a way for an organism to use characteristics like taste to avoid toxic or infectious foods in the future. I would even propose that this phenomenon is well known to careless drinkers who, after having overindulged in their youth in a certain alcoholic beverage, can later on not smell, taste, or even think about the drink without experiencing the same suffering that struck them the day after the party. Taste aversion can last a long time. Every time turnip purée was served in my school cafeteria, I spent the entire lunch break trying to force myself to eat it without it coming up again, and did not realize that this conditioned nausea might have entitled me to a doctor's note certifying that I did not tolerate this famous Swedish dish. I had presumably at some point become ill after eating turnip purée, maybe for a completely unrelated reason, but the perception that this dish was dangerous was firmly imprinted in the body for many years.

But back to Ader's rats. The rats were exposed to cyclophosphamide, a substance that not only made them nauseous but that is also harmful to white blood cells. Rats exposed to the sweet taste several times after being conditioned to cyclophosphamide appeared to die more often than rats who had not coupled the taste to the toxic substance. The control rats had been exposed to the same amounts and dosages of both cyclophosphamide and sugar solution as the conditioned rats, but not in a systematic order that allowed them to be associated with one other.

Ader hypothesized that the death of the conditioned rats could be due to a conditioned depression of the white blood cells that weakened the rats' immunity and thus their resilience. In that case, the sweet taste would have become a conditioned stimulus: a reliable signal of the drug. After becoming a conditioned stimulus, the taste could then in itself be sufficient to start physiological reactions similar to the drug. This speculation was later shown through high-quality research studies to be true, and countless variations of the phenomenon have been proven using Pavlov's rigorous research methods. Bob Ader later explained that one reason he thought along these lines of conditioning was that he, as a psychologist, was totally ignorant of immunology. He did not "know" that the immune system regulated itself without the involvement of the nervous system— the prevailing view at the time. Nor did Ader know that Russian scientists had been on the same track in the beginning of the century.

A currently active researcher, who is also a great outside-of-the-box thinker, is the German professor Manfred Schedlowski. While it is unlikely that this fact is related to his habit of riding a Harley Davidson with his substantial moustache blowing in the breeze, let us assume it is for the sake of entertainment and illustration. Schedlowski's research puts the conditioned immune responses into a placebo perspective. He does this to see how important healing processes can be affected by behavior in both an automatic and unconscious way. Schedlowski's many experiments on conditioning have included hands-on tests to determine if the effects can also affect clinically relevant biological processes. Schedlowski tried to use classical conditioning to suppress the immunological processes that cause transplanted organs to be rejected, and tested this method with heart transplantations! Luckily, Schedlowski is not eccentric enough to try this technique on humans, but instead uses a well-established model in which an extra heart is transplanted into a rat. Luckily for humans, one might add.

The extra heart works and beats for some time before being rejected by a powerful immune response, unless the so-called T-cell activity is depressed by a substance called Cyclosporin A. This is the same substance used to counteract the rejection of new organs, such as a kidney or liver, in humans. Schedlowski conditioned this potent drug to a sweet taste, and with the help of this taste and a tiny amount of Cyclosporin A, the survival of the transplanted heart was clearly prolonged. About one fifth of the rats that were conditioned did not reject the new heart at all, and the others accepted it for a longer period of time compared to rats who received the same substances but in the wrong order. Thus, the difference was that the sugar solution given to the control rats did *not* act as a reliable signal (a conditioned stimulus) for the active drug, so that learning did not occur. In other words, we are back to *prediction*, referring to the tendency of the nervous system to try to predict events so that reactions can begin in time. But now I have to correct myself, because I have just shown that the same tendency applies to the immune system, and of course to the other systems that make our bodies work—the tendency of the *organism* to want to predict events. But of course, the nervous system is the master of this game and would win any body championship. In second place is probably the immune system, which is also extremely malleable and adaptable. Schedlowski's organ rejection experiments have been replicated several times, and some of the underlying mechanisms have been elucidated.

Conditioning is surely a form of expectation, and conscious expectation—like the example of expecting to become nauseous from turnip purée—can, of course, also depend on conditioning. However, dividing placebo mechanisms into the two main classes of expectation and conditioning is still useful, and summarizes two different key principles underlying the placebo phenomenon. From the perspective of this book, we learn two important things from the aforementioned example: how important top-down phenomena are in controlling physiological systems, and that the control can involve a system central for our health—the immune system—a system that is active both in the brain and throughout the body.

A final question arises before we leave the topic of placebos, namely, who is inclined and easily influenced enough to let their bodies be controlled in this way by psychological processes? The answer is that everyone is, even if it is difficult to predict exactly who will react and to what extent at a certain occasion. In fact, we know relatively little about sensitivity to placebos, even though we know that not everyone will respond with a placebo reaction every time. Given the rule that the placebo effect utilizes several general principles for predicting events and activating physiological processes, and that contextual factors play a role, it is perhaps not surprising that the range of variation is so great. The idea of being gullible, and thus sensitive to placebos, can therefore be discarded.

In the summer of 2013, I hosted a scientific conference in Stockholm, and one afternoon I had booked a boat that picked up our group after a reception in the city hall, where two of our guests had previously enjoyed the big Nobel Prize Banquet after being awarded the prize for their respective research accomplishments. We boarded the boat right outside the city hall and were able to enjoy an idyllic Swedish summer day that exploded with joy. I headed for the bar and bought some beers for myself and Bruce Beutler, who received the 2011 Nobel Prize in Physiology or Medicine for his discoveries about the immune system, which I will return to later. After several more visits to the bar, the party atmosphere grew considerably, and the conversation flowed easily, as it can under the insidious influence of alcohol. I thought it would be best not to drink one of our honored guests under the table, but decided that one last round couldn't hurt. I then discovered, to my surprise (I was going to write "alarm," but perhaps that would give the wrong impression) that I had bought non-alcoholic beer. The atmosphere, the boat trip, the weather—everything certainly contributed to the party feeling, together with the conditioning (the taste of beer as a signal for an alcoholic beverage) and a conscious expectation based on my knowledge of how many times I ran to the bar and felt cold beer in my hands. I shared my discovery with Beutler, who is as close as you can come to a legitimately talented person, who was also completely unaware that we were drunk on placebo beer. We got off at The Museum of Modern Art, where, I have to admit, we went directly to the bar and each ordered an ordinary beer (= alcohol + placebo) before we settled down at the outdoor cafe.

When brain damage distorts body perception

If we claim that the brain constructs an idea of the body, and that we can demonstrate this with a combination of logic, rubber hands, deception, extra hearts, Noble Prize winners, and Barbie dolls, then there must also be patients with brain injuries suffering from syndromes where body perception is distorted, right? Brain imaging studies of healthy individuals are fantastic, but if we also study patients suffering from debilitating brain damage, we can achieve even deeper knowledge of how the brain understands the body. Functional loss that affects your own body is, in my opinion, particularly tragic and enigmatic because the way we experience our bodies is so close to how we perceive ourselves. We are now tiptoeing around the knowledge needed to understand the physical basis of our identity. Who are you when the image of your own body drifts far beyond the limits of what is reasonable? Neuropsychological phenomena and case studies are infinitely interesting, but I'll limit myself to a few short examples that show once again how even the experience of the body is not a direct reflection of true reality. We experience the body based on a calculation that the brain does on more or less sound grounds.[3]

A person suffering from *anosognosia* may deny that there is anything wrong with a body part, which may be paralysed after a stroke, despite a doctor's direct request to try to show that they can move it. In *somatoparaphrenia*—a more extreme variant—the patient denies that a body part is even their own, claiming that it belongs to another person. These syndromes may occur in *hemispatial neglect*, which is not uncommon after a stroke. In this syndrome, a patient may fail to pay attention to or interact with the part of their environment located opposite the damaged half of the brain. The condition is most common after injuries to the right lobe, and difficulties arise when it comes to things happening to the left

---

[3] The American neurologist Oliver Sacks has written several fascinating books describing remarkable functional failures in patients, many of which concern body perception. In *A leg to stand on* (1984) he describes how he himself was affected after an accident, when his injured leg no longer felt like a part of his body.

of the person, or to the left part of an object that is to be attended to. The odd part is that the condition can also apply to one's own body, so that a patient only combs the hair on one side of the head or shaves half the face. Half of the body disappears in some way, and it becomes very difficult for the patient to let the light of consciousness shine over the left part of the body. When neglect applies to one's own body rather than to a part of the outside world, it is called *personal neglect*. A reminiscent phenomenon is the *alien hand syndrome* in which a hand is experienced as having a life of its own, doing things directly against the will of what you would call the legitimate owner of the hand. For example, the insubordinate hand might try to slap, punch, or undress the owner, in spite of the opposite hand trying to stop it.

It seems with these types of conditions that the necessary updating of the body parts' position and condition and the ability to focus on them does not work properly. Another kind of dysfunction after a brain injury can rather relate to one's knowledge about how the body is composed and interrelationships between the body parts. In a condition called *autotopagnosia*, patients are unable to point out their own body parts, even though they can identify other objects on request and manage similar tasks that do not apply to their own bodies. Perhaps one can say that they lack a strong concept of the body's structure, rather than a concept of the body's condition.

Injuries to the posterior insula are generally associated with how interoceptive information is represented—such as changes in how pain, temperature, or touch are experienced—but are also associated with anosognosia. Damage to the anterior insula is more often associated with emotional disturbances that affect how one experiences the body. It should be noted, however, that surgical procedures in the insula do not necessarily produce significant effects or lead to clear problems. Damage to the anterior cingulum has been associated, for example, with changes in how pain is experienced so that one can feel but not care about pain or discomfort.

I constantly return to the fact that what we experience as the body is a calculation, or an approximate compilation of information. That claim may seem a bit trivial. How could one even experience a body without a brain? And does it not have to assemble different types of information to create a representation of something, whether it is the outside world or the state of your own body? The point is that extreme cases of illusions or strange neurological phenomena show that different aspects of body perception can be manipulated or disturbed. The examples also show that perception of the body and its health status is built up in parts and assembled, even constructed, into a coherent view. It is in this way that we experience a very central component of our health, and perhaps nothing is more important to humans than our perception of health.

That is why attention, expectations, and internal explanatory models play a role in our health assessment, and why psychological knowledge is so important for strengthening health and treating ill health. Psychology is a central but often overlooked framework for understanding and improving health. What are the effects in today's society of widespread health consumerism—with health as a central commodity—on our ability to stay healthy? Or to feel healthy? We have internal defence systems that send information about the body's condition, also on the tiny scale of microbes, to the brain. Research about these signals and the roles they play in emotions and behavior continues to grow exponentially.

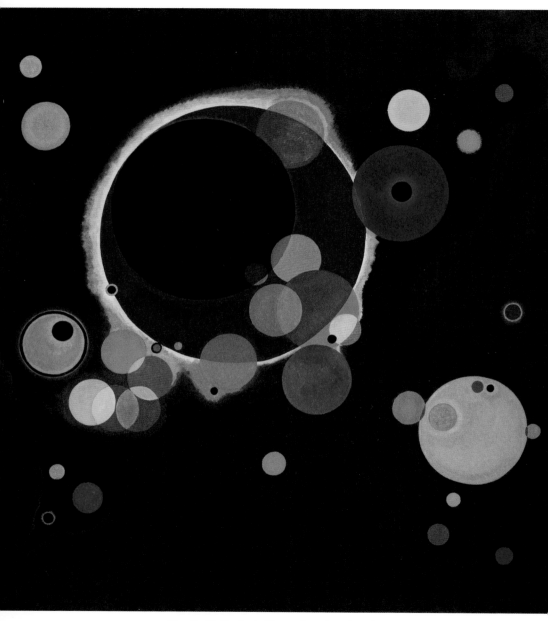

Vassily Kadinsky's "Several circles" (1926)

3

OUR INNER DEFENSE SYSTEMS

A war is taking place on and in your body at this very moment—you are under attack. Large amounts of foreign organisms exist on and in your body; some are dangerous and need to be neutralized. The battle between the body's own cells and foreign organisms takes place at the microscopic level and, for the most part, you are not aware of the myriads of organisms trying to take part in the attractive reproductive environment your body offers. But when the immune system decides to react forcefully, you begin to feel sick, since the brain senses the inflammation that is launched during the body's counterattack.

The immune system's job description

Not all microorganisms are harmful, and many are a prerequisite for good health. This applies to different kinds of bacteria that populate the gastrointestinal tract. It is a difficult trade-off for the immune system to determine when a part of your body is damaged and should be aided by the body's cleaning crew. It may apply to older obsolete cells, or even to tumor cells that are, after all, parts of the body, albeit potentially dangerous ones. Therefore these trade-offs between self and non-self, and between dangerous and harmless, pose a risk of ill health when the reactions are not directed against the proper targets, do not happen with the right force, or even fail to take place at all. Even though you would be at risk of dying from brushing your teeth without your immune

The Inflamed Feeling. Mats Lekander, Oxford University Press. © Mats Lekander 2022.
DOI: 10.1093/oso/9780198863441.003.0003

cells,[1] too strong a reaction, such as sepsis or allergic shock, or a cytokine storm in response to a coronavirus, can kill you. Several of the points in this book are based on the immune system and its communication with the brain. I will therefore give an overview of the immune system's structure and the fascinating protective activity that is constantly taking place in our bodies.

The cells of the immune system, the white blood cells, are spread throughout the body in the lymphatic system (lymph nodes, lymph vessels, and some organs such as the spleen), the blood, and other tissues. White blood cells also reside in brain tissue. A foreign organism that enters the body must first be able to bypass chemical and mechanical barriers including the skin and mucous membranes, among others. Once it has entered, it can be detected by the white blood cells, which then communicate in a very intricate way in order to initiate a counterattack. The substance they detect and that generates a counterattack is called an antigen; the antigen does not in fact need to be an invading microorganism but can also be cells in your own body. Moreover, dust particles, debris, or the wooden sliver that got stuck in your foot when you dove off from a pier, belong to the same category of enemies that your immune system attacks.

Innate immunity

The fastest part of the immune system is the innate immune system. It is called *innate* because it is with us from birth and works in a similar way throughout life. *Granulocytes* and *macrophages* are important cells in the innate branch of the immune system and they react, inter alia, by "eating up" (phagocyte) foreign substances or harmful cells. Accordingly, macrophage means "big eater." Another task these cells perform is making the

---

[1] If we imagine that during toothbrushing you make a wound in the gums, so that infectious agents can sneak in.

site of the injury or attack available and attractive to other cells. When the inflammatory response is initiated, for example at the site of the annoying sliver stubbornly lodged in your toe, it is part of this same process. At the site of the inflammation, fluid builds up, cells accumulate, and their various products are secreted in large quantities.

The innate immune system and its cells are developmentally very old and are similarly constructed in everything from simple molluscs to great apes. In fact, your sick dog—or even your sick snail, if you belong to the minute group of snail owners—responds with similar mechanisms at the beginning of an infection, and displays behavioral changes that I will return to later. During my doctoral studies, when I first began working in the lab with white blood cells, I could not believe my eyes when I learned to distinguish "eating" blood cells from other cells. My laboratory mentor, Marja Hallström, gave me the following instructions: "Pour iron filings into your test tube and let the cells you want to get rid of eat the iron fragments. Then hold a magnet against the bottom of the test tube when you pour the remaining non-magnetic ones into another test tube." At the time I thought she might be playing a practical joke on the newcomer—and an unsuspecting psychology student at that—but it in fact worked exactly as she had described. I found the method to be incredibly low-tech, even back in the now so distant early 1990s.

The innate immune system plays a key role in quickly starting a counterattack, but at least two other aspects are also important. The innate response acts as a link to the so-called acquired immune system, so that a more specific response can be organized and future protection can be built up. But for even more effective protection, an additional defense system needs to be involved, and what could be more suitable than sending signals to the body's superhero, the brain? This is something that macrophages are particularly good at; you can look forward to learning more in Chapter 4 about what happens when the brain receives these important signals. But one thing at a time—back to immunity.

Acquired immunity

After phagocytosis (when immune cells swallow foreign substances), the macrophage presents a small fragment of the processed material to another group of white blood cells, the *lymphocytes*. The lymphocytes are evolutionarily newer and have been added to older systems within the vertebrate immune system. The principle here is specificity, so that a specific pathogen can be precisely identified when the macrophage has presented it to the lymphocytes. This differs from the way in which the innate immune system works—a system based on general recognition, for example, of substances that occur in many types of bacteria.

If a specific antigen is recognized by a lymphocyte with the proper receptors, the lymphocyte begins to divide rapidly. These cells have receptors that only fit with the particular infectious agent, and not with any other. Despite extensive expansion, it takes several days before the number of cells is large enough. During this time, the body must rely on the innate branch of the immune system.

After contact with an antigen is completed—when the infection is over—a number of lymphocytes with these exact receptors remain for future use, that is, if we should be exposed to the infectious agent again. We have then become immune, and may not even notice when we have been exposed to the same substance before the specific immune system has done its job. A targeted attack means that great general activation, and accompanying feelings, are not needed. As is probably apparent, this is the principle behind vaccination: to intentionally create an immunological memory so that lymphocytes with the right receptors can quickly strike against a particular intruder the next time we encounter it.

Some lymphocytes are called B-cells and produce antibodies—exportable receptors that match specific antigens and that can cause all kinds of misery for an intruder. If the intruder enters a native cell, which viruses must do in order to survive and multiply, the antibodies are not effective.

In that case, other lymphocytes (so-called cytotoxic T-cells) and natural killer (NK) cells are needed to attack. The NK cells are actually fundamental in the innate branch of the immune system, but thus also play an important role in acquired immunity. Antibodies can then control exactly which cells should taste the NK cells' toxic kiss of death when it is nearby. The antibody-directed portion of the immune system is called humoral (fluid-related) because the antibodies are transported in the body's fluid system. The branch in which kisses of death are distributed in direct contact with other cells is called cellular or cell-mediated. These two branches of the immune system, the humoral and the cellular, must be activated by other cells, which happens, for example, when they come into contact with antigens.

This is all fine and well, that is, if it works as it should. Many diseases result when the activation process does not work properly, such as allergies or autoimmune diseases. The immune system's target then becomes harmless substances, such as pollen, or important bodily organs, such as insulin-producing cells (in Type 1 diabetes) or nerve cells (in multiple sclerosis). The result is too much activity against the wrong target, where substances or body cells that should be recognized but not reacted to, are unfortunately not only recognized but also attacked. Substances that regulate how active other cells should be are produced, for example, by T-helper cells or macrophages in the innate immune system. Many of the released substances are used to slow down and limit the level of immunological activity.

Friendly bacteria

In the preface, I described how activities in the body can make you want to behave differently, and that parasites' efforts to multiply also can make them try to change your behavior for their benefit. Most cells found in the human body are not at all human, but rather bacteria. The genes that selfishly struggle to survive in your body are, to a negligible degree, your own—a majority actually belong to microorganisms. So, you are a minority within yourself.

This may sound intimidating, but peaceful coexistence and even mutual exchange with these microorganisms is the norm. In fact, they are an important part of our overall immune system. These microorganisms play a role in stimulating and training our white blood cells so that they develop properly. But the microorganisms we carry with us from an early age also fight off foreign organisms that threaten to infect us. In this process, organisms in our inner world can even secrete their own type of antibiotic to fight an intruder.

In recent decades, our internal environment of microorganisms seems to have changed. Increased antibiotic use, caesarean sections instead of vaginal delivery, and various lifestyle factors are believed to have contributed to a limited flora of microorganisms compared to how it was during previous generations. Many researchers are investigating whether this change is linked to substantial health changes we have seen during the same period. The incidence of certain conditions has increased greatly, including asthma, allergies, diabetes, and obesity.

Regulating the activity of the immune system

When the immune system is activated, the white blood cells release substances aimed at communicating with other cells and regulating their activities. An important class of such substances is *cytokines*—hormone-like proteins that act over short distances (on immune cells next to or even on the same cell that released the substance) or longer distances. It is well described how these cytokines affect a number of cells and how they regulate processes in the body. But a lesser known fact is that the brain is one of the important targets, and here we are approaching the heart of the matter. As will be seen, the cytokines are active in many processes other than purely immunological ones, and they play a key role in the interaction between the nervous and immune systems. When I wrote my student thesis and began doctoral studies at the Karolinska Hospital and Karolinska Institutet cancer clinic, I learned a great lot from an experienced immunologist named Henric Blomgren. Henric predicted that I would become Sweden's first professor of psychoneuroimmunology, but that I would *not* achieve that goal by working with cytokines, which, by the early 1990s, had come into fashion in immunology. His first prediction ultimately came true, but I did not take his advice on the cytokines. By then, a large number of cytokines of different "families" had been discovered, but which were, to be on the safe side, known to the scientific public by many alternative names. Sure, one could feel confused for less.

When the cytokine people get started with their enumerations, Henric said, it is impossible to follow along, and no one has a clue how these molecules are connected to one another or what they really do. Curiosity about these difficult-to-understand cytokines was nevertheless great and would only increase during the 1990s and spread far beyond immunology. They would even spark the interest of other professional groups such as endocrinologists, neurologists, and, it turned out, psychologists. An eye-opening article I read on the subject was called "Cytokines for psychologists" and described both the relevance of the cytokines to behavior and the role of behavior in the immune system. In particular, one of the cytokines, Interleukin (IL)-1, had already been shown to affect the brain.

A colleague at Karolinska Institutet shared a surprising anecdote with me. They went on a trip to Cuba and met Fidel Castro himself. During an unguarded moment, Castro took the colleague aside and said, "Tell me *h*everything you know about Inter*h*eleukin-1!" Castro admittedly accused the United States of having spread dengue fever in Cuba. But perhaps his question about IL-1 was not based on an interest in biological warfare and its effect on the brain, but rather on the major investment in biotechnology and immunology that Castro had made.[2]

---

[2] One of the cytokines that affect the brain, Interferon-alpha, is used to treat certain cancers and some infections. When the rumor about interferon as a potential cure for cancer spread in the 1980s, the microbiology enthusiast Castro thought that this was something that

The immune system's complex processing of information, its communication, regulation of other systems, and, not least, ability to form memories remind us of the nervous system. Due to the commonalities between the immune and nervous systems, it is clear that many challenges can be better addressed through their mutual communication and collaboration. The problems are often similar and, to a large extent, deal with risk assessment.

Two defense systems with a common goal

If you look back at the description earlier in the chapter of how the immune system works, you'll see great similarities with tasks that are important for the central nervous system. Like the immune system, the nervous system should recognize harmful organisms and situations and make difficult adjustments to protect one's own life and that of one's offspring. It must be flexible and adapted over time to the environment in which you live. In a dangerous situation, a number of fast and partly pre-programmed response patterns must be launched, but they must also adapt to the current situation. This involves control and regulation of a genetically predetermined activity, which is also fine-tuned and influenced by learning during the time as a fetus, after birth, throughout childhood, and during exposure to all sorts of dangers. The immune system should recognize dangerous substances, just as we do in the outside world through vision, hearing, smell, taste, and sensation. The total weight of the white blood cells, about 1.5 kilograms, corresponds to the weight of the brain, and the cells are scattered in an intricate network throughout the body. So the question then arises, would it be effective for the systems to cooperate? If we accept that assumption—with the support of innumerable research

Cuba should also have. A house on the outskirts of Havana was turned into a laboratory, and after 42 days they succeeded in producing interferon after working non-stop on the task. Castro visited the laboratory every day to monitor the project's progress.

reports and logical arguments—one conclusion is obvious: what we do and feel could affect our health and our ability to defend ourselves against illness, and our internal defense systems would be able to influence what we know, do, and think.

Fact or fiction: Stress, sleep, and health

In addition to the research on how immune responses can be modified by learning through conditioning, an important research area within psycho-neuroimmunology has been about stress. Why waste time on this when everyone knows that stress is harmful to the immune system? Well, because it is not really true, and because the answer to the question—when will we ever learn?—is so much more complex than one would initially believe. We know that severe long-term stress depresses many of the immune system's functions, but does this make us sick (or even healthier)? Not necessarily. Since health is associated with properly balanced activity in the immune system, it is not clear whether increased or decreased activity is good or bad for a particular person and a particular disease. Too much activity in any part of the immune system not only increases the risk of ill health through faulty regulation, which can surface as an allergy or auto-immune disease, but also the risk of *feeling* ill and behaving in a disadvantageous way. It can even, it is believed, increase the risk of mental illness.

Overall, the body of research shows that long and severe stress is associated with a greater risk of ill health.[3] But remember that the effects are not necessarily large, and that one advantage, compared to many other risk factors (for example, genetic conditions, certain environmental factors,

---

[3] A caveat about this research: since knowledge of stress and health over the long term is based on observations rather than experiments, knowledge about causation is still uncertain. Exactly what it is that increases the risk of ill health following long-term exposure to severe stress is often unclear; in many cases, there is probably also a reverse causal relationship. This means that factors related to health and disease affect one's subjective stress level and can explain some of the connections frequently found between stress and health.

physical injuries), is that stress can be modified by the individual. It is not easy to change one's lifestyle, but it is doable. For many, treating potential sleep problems, physical activity, and other methods that counteract long-term stress are achievable changes, and one can at least avoid systematically neglecting these behaviors. If you cannot change your stress exposures, then it is comforting to know that many other factors also affect your actual long-term health. The negative effects of stress on the brain and health are often exaggerated by the media, stress consultants, and lecturers. The stress system has of course been developed to keep us alive, not to kill us. This is clear when studying how stress affects the immune system, as the acute stress response stimulates immune cells to enhance protection and performance in times of danger. And it is these acute effects that we know most about.

If I was given the task of designing a defense system that would capture acute threats of physical injury, such as those faced by an ill-fated human being, what would I include? Let's begin the thought experiment with the nervous and hormonal systems: Predict a threat at the first sign of trouble and then quickly initiate a response? Check. Make energy available to the major muscle groups to support fight or flight? Check. Reduce pain sensitivity? Check. Sharpen your attention and focus on the danger? Check. Support memory encoding to be used in future similar situations? Check. We then proceed with the immune system: Suppress the immune system to prioritize other defense mechanisms and then rev it up if it seems necessary? Hardly.

Dangerous situations entail increased risk of injury and infection. Shouldn't the immune system be required to heal wounds and manage infection which, with some luck, are the only consequences of the hostile encounter? We would therefore include a function that enables the alarm response (stress) to *activate* the immune system. The cells should be prepared and several of them should choose to swim around in the blood so they can quickly reach the body part in need of attention. Fortunately, this is also the case. Acute stress means that the innate part of the immune system, which is already fast, is put on alert awaiting further information. To use a military analogy, the soldiers (the white blood cells) are found primarily in their barracks (spleen and other organs), but when danger arises, they patrol the roads (the bloodstream) in greater numbers in order to quickly reach the battlefield (the site of the damage after the attack) if necessary. There are also basic learning functions so that well-balanced attacks can be directed in a safe and energy-efficient way the next time the same threat arises. The threat thus leads to similar changes in the immune system as it does in the nervous and hormone systems: increased energy, "attention," and memory encoding.

So most of the functions of the nervous system thought experiment also apply to the immune system. The immune system should also regulate its own functional level and protect the body by activating survival networks corresponding to the prevailing threat level. The functional similarities are reasonable for two systems that monitor internal and external hazards. It is no surprise then that the systems cooperate to such an extent that it is sometimes difficult or even impossible to distinguish between them. The acute stress response to vaccination increases the immune response and enhances memory function. This is similar to how it works with fear, where the emotional response effectively enhances the encoding of memory. So if you have small children and find it uncomfortable to see them cry when they get a vaccination shot, you can comfort yourself with the idea that the pain may help activate the immune system and strengthen the encoding of the immunological memory. On the other hand, your child will likely remember the nasty syringe better than the subsequent ice cream.

Acute stress increases the activity of the innate part of the immune system, and we know this from a variety of research on both animals and humans. Acquired immunity is less influenced by acute stress but takes a beating following long-term stress. By "take a beating," I mean that its functions, needed for a balanced and fine-tuned counterattack, can be suppressed or disturbed.

An example of how stress that lasts for several weeks affects health can be illustrated through the common cold. Various experiments, many of which were conducted by the American researcher Sheldon Cohen, have shown that the risk of catching a common cold is higher during periods of high stress. In Cohen's experiments, healthy volunteers inhaled cold viruses; the researchers then measured the degree to which the individuals actually caught a cold (remember that not everyone is infected or equally affected when exposed to a virus). The subjects' stress levels during the previous weeks and months were measured via questionnaires: the stronger and more prolonged the reported stress prior to the experiment, the higher the risk of catching a cold when exposed to the virus. Similar studies with research animals have also shown that when stress levels are actively manipulated, so that one has experimental control over exposure both to the microorganisms and stress, the results of the human studies were confirmed. Perhaps you are now wondering if it is true that the risk of getting a cold is particularly high right *after* a long period of intense work, like when a work season is over and a holiday begins? It would be easy for me to say that it is not true . . . but I don't think I can. The answer is that it could be true, but that we simply don't know. It is unfortunately not easy to investigate, and people's memories of this happening do not always reflect the objective truth.

Similarly, length of sleep has in some few studies also been linked to the risk of catching a cold—the less sleep time before virus exposure, the greater the risk of infection. The underlying mechanisms behind these relationships are not well understood, but appear to be related to dysregulation of the immune system after stress hormones have been active for several weeks. One effect of the dysregulation is the increased production of substances that tell the brain you are sick.

Let's move on to how white blood cells send messages to the brain about your state of health and how they make you long for your bed. Okay, maybe you're already feeling that way, so I'll modify that last sentence and instead write, long *even more* for your bed. As I write this on an early summer morning, I'm half lying on a couch in a summer cottage; when I stop to think about it, I could easily go back to bed and quickly fall asleep. But I feel quite healthy and can probably resist the temptation. But with a greater sense of physical malaise, I would definitely go back to bed and pull down not only the physical but also the intellectual blinds. The fact that my young son, deeply absorbed in an old Donald Duck book, just nestled up to me, increases my motivation to stay awake. Motivation affects what we want and what we choose to do, and, cunningly, the immune system is excellent at manipulating our motivation to get what it needs.

The brain can both stimulate and inhibit the activity of white blood cells. During acute stress, inflammatory activity is stimulated, while some functions are depressed or disturbed during longer-term stress. For example, certain hormones that are associated with stress are utilized in the brain's control of the immune system. In Figure 3.1 we see cortisol, which has different effects on the immune system depending on the levels. Substances such as norepinephrine and epinephrine can also affect the white blood cells, as can acetylcholine. The control can be executed either by the hormones circulating in the blood (dashed lines in Figure 3.1) or by close contact resembling synapses between nerves (solid lines in Figure 3.1) and white blood cells. If you remember the anecdote

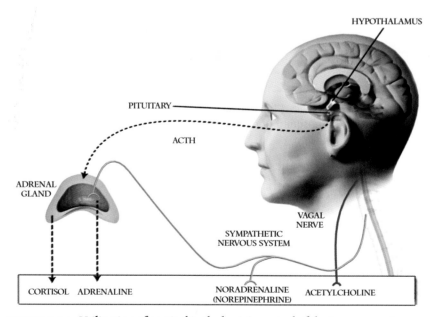

FIGURE 3.1 Utilization of cortisol in the brain's control of the immune system.

Mats Lekander and Rasmus Pettersson. Adaptation from Alllergi i praxis 3/2008, Mats Lekander and Caroline Olgart Höglund

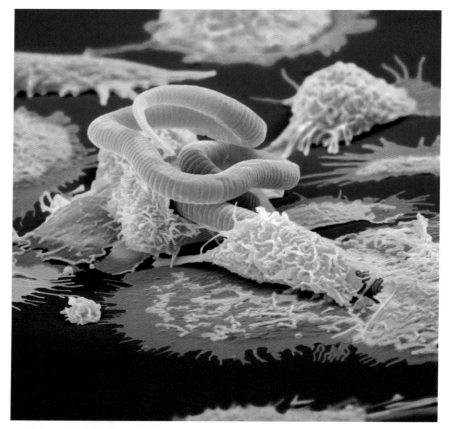

FIGURE 3.2 Macrophages ("big eaters") attacking a parasitic larva spread from human to human via mosquito, and which can cause elephantiasis.

from the preface, it was the communication between the nervous system and the immune system that I described and became so fascinated by during the interview methodology exercise.

Macrophages (see Figure 3.2) are good at secreting cytokines that act as signals within the immune system and that also inform the brain when they encounter micro-level threats. The same substances can be secreted in the brain by similar cells when they receive messages from within the body.

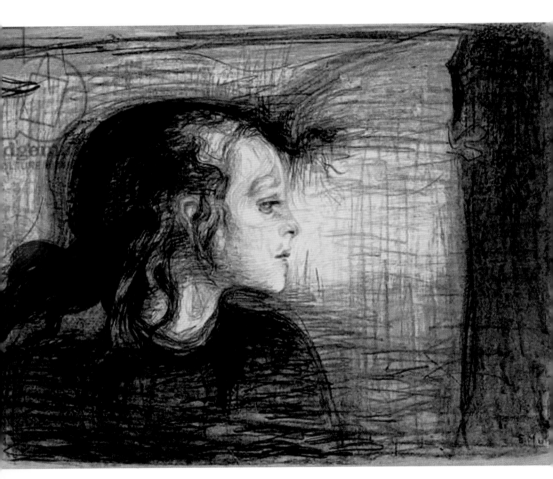

Edvard Munch's "The sick girl" [Det syke barn] (1896)

4

THE SICKNESS RESPONSE

The next time you hear yourself say, "I don't feel good, I think I'll go back to bed," you will know why you are saying it—the immune system has taken control of your brain. Machinery passed along to you via your ancestors' genes is activated and makes you want to rest. Your ancestors speak to you, so to say, through this feeling. A specific series of electrical and chemical impulses has been triggered and makes you think of only one thing: lying down and being still. In the short term, it sounds great that the body adapts, making you want to rest and reduce your activity when you are ill. But when you think about this for a while, an unpleasant thought comes to mind: Can this system become "locked" and stay active over a longer period of time while you remain passive without fully engaging in everyday life? Can it be activated without a specific threat, when the perceived danger is not real, but is the consequence of—you guessed it—sustained activation of your defense system?

Think about how it felt the last time you had a serious cold or flu. I would wager that you recall feeling a little depressed, and perhaps a bit worried or anxious. Without a doubt, you felt fatigued and even felt some degree of pain. It is also not unlikely that a wish to keep to yourself will appear on your mental list. These kinds of reactions are triggered when danger arises, especially when your body is threatened from within at the micro level. The receptors that notice danger somewhere in the body were called "the eyes of the immune system" by Bruce Beutler (the Nobel laureate I referred to during the placebo intoxication on non-alcoholic beer story). He discovered the receptor that recognizes a typical fragment found in the wall of a relevant cell. This small molecule within the bacterium is called

The Inflamed Feeling. Mats Lekander, Oxford University Press. © Mats Lekander 2022.
DOI: 10.1093/oso/9780198863441.003.0004

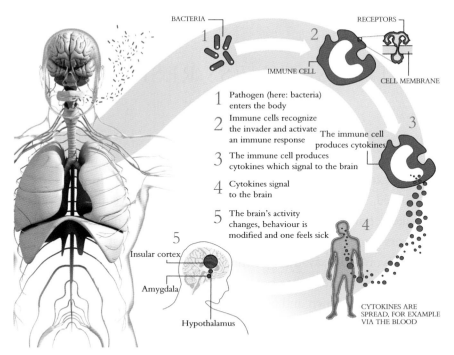

FIGURE 4.1 A schematic illustration of the sickness response. Receptors on the macrophage recognize a tiny part of the bacterium called lipopolysaccharide or endotoxin, which starts the sickness response.

Mats Lekander, Caroline Olgart Höglund and Bianka Karshikoff. Image: David Nyman

endotoxin (or lipopolysaccharide) and acts as a flag or ID marker that the immune system uses to identify the bacterium (see Figures 4.1 and 4.2).

As I'll describe in more detail later on, both the power and timing of an immunological reaction can be modified by the brain as it seeks to predict the future and guess what should happen next. It may seem surprising that external information, contexts, and guesses can affect the strength of a reaction in the body, but this fact actually aligns the reaction with that of other normal physiological systems. Although the innate immune response to infection is highly conserved (it is similar across species, is inherited, and has changed very little over time), the power of the reaction is modified based on the context. Since that's the brain's normal modus operandi, why should it be any different for disease reactions?

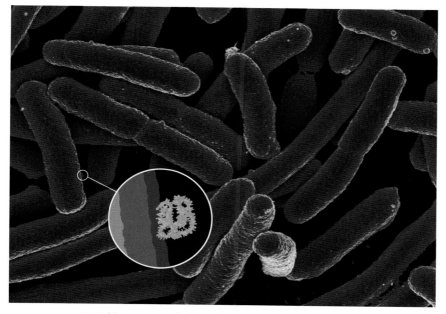

FIGURE 4.2 E. *Coli* bacteria, with the endotoxin molecule (inset) corresponding to a flag or ID card to the immune system.

Rasmus Pettersson. Image: Sciencephoto

The phenomenon itself is called functional flexibility. A congenital response pattern must be able to be regulated by the context.

Your behavior (and that of other animals) when sick

When the immune system is activated, for example during an infection, signal products are released that reach the brain. These products are called cytokines, and have interested and baffled immunologists, endocrinologists, neurologists, psychologists, and even dictators (according to my story in Chapter 3). Cytokines are, as I said, a kind of protein with hormone-like properties. They can stimulate specific white blood cells to divide and multiply, increase or decrease immunological activity, make cells more or less aggressive, stimulate the production of antibodies, and much more. When cytokines were discovered in the 1970s, they were thought to be confined to the immune system, but soon it became clear that they are quite similar to other substances in the body, and are also part of the language spoken by the nervous and hormone systems. Because the substances play an important role when one system tries to regulate the other, as when the immune system tells the brain "slow down, go to bed," these cytokines are often examined when researchers look for connections between psychological phenomena and health.

Through a clever communication system, the cytokines affect the brain, which interprets them (with a simplified but functionally correct description) as signs of sickness. We feel tired, feverish, and depressed, our bodies ache, and we may not want to do more than lie down under a warm blanket. We experience pain as worse than usual. The effects depend on the immune system's ability to influence the brain and the rest of the nervous system. This pattern of changes is called sickness behavior, or a sickness response. But is this behavioral pattern surprising, considering that one is sick and thus in a weakened state? An organism that is in a weakened state should simply not be able to move and behave as normal. What is interesting is that the sickness response described here represents a state of *motivation*, the goal of which is to make us want to behave in a way that is advantageous, given our current state, in order to improve our odds. This link between a threat to our survival, a certain physiological response, and a propensity to exhibit certain behaviors is very similar to how human emotions, such as joy or anger, work. We will return to this in Chapter 7. I will then argue that the sickness response is in fact an emotion, among others, but one that has been missed by the psychologists and neuroscientists. But now, back to how we behave when we become sick.

The sickness response:

- Fatigue, increased need for sleep
- Depressed mood, increased anxiety, and worry
- Reduced appetite
- Increased sensitivity to pain
- Reduced interest in social interaction

An increased body temperature during a fever makes it difficult for some contagious agents to multiply. There are also other benefits of a higher body temperature when you are ill, as long as the fever is kept within reasonable limits. But it is costly to increase body temperature—every degree of increase involves a significant cost to metabolism. For support, behavior can be modified to conserve energy.

We want to sleep and rest to increase the chance of surviving an infection that caused an immune reaction, and not just because we are weakened by disease. Because we feel cold, we want to keep warm and not waste too much energy increasing our body temperature and supporting the fever response. When we lose our appetite, we do not want to go out in a weakened state searching for food; at the same time, we avoid feeding the bacteria. Because we feel less inclined to social interaction, we do not invest energy in meeting other people. We focus on our inner world and on the symptoms we feel, such as pain or other body discomfort. This makes us slow down, and overall, it improves our odds of healing.

Thus, when the body responds to illness, our feelings and behaviors change. In the short term, this seems to be a good strategy to promote our natural healing mechanisms.[1] But in the longer term, if the reaction doesn't shut itself down, it is not such a good thing—a subject I'll return to.

How your immune system communicates with your brain

Immunology used to have a reputation for being the last outpost of the classical biomedical paradigm in such a way that brain function, behavior, and social processes were considered to be irrelevant. The immune system is undoubtedly highly capable of functioning on its own, and the most peculiar and complicated processes can indeed be studied in test tubes.

---

[1] We can be certain that the strategy was good for our ancestors, but we cannot know for sure how good the strategy is for us today, in our present living conditions.

But if this is the case, why bother involving the brain and branches of the nervous system when it is already so complex and capable? The view of the brain as an immunologically privileged organ (a place that the immune system cannot access) has given way over recent years, but it has taken an astonishing amount of time. In any case, the tools used by immune and nerve cells to communicate with one another have existed since ancient times, and of course long before the artificial boundaries of science and its diverse subdisciplines made it difficult for us to think in a system perspective, or about the interactions among functional systems with unclear boundaries.

Imagine a simple mollusc such as a snail, with clusters of neural cells rather than a brain in the strict sense. In these animals, immune cells cooperate with nerve cells to organize a defense against infection and tissue damage. When similar animals arose more than 500 million years ago, collaboration between such neighboring cells was a prerequisite. When organisms with separate and protected brains developed, there was a need for the body's immune system to send signals to the brain (and vice versa), but with the aggravating fact that a blood-brain barrier (tightly interconnected cells protecting the brain and preventing, or making it difficult for, substances and cells to pass through) stood in the way. Since communication between neural and immune functions was important for survival, several different communication pathways arose to cross the blood-brain barrier. These mechanisms are partially documented. One pathway for neural-immune system communication is based on the movement of signalling substances, such as cytokines, through the bloodstream to cells at the blood-brain barrier. These cells are then activated, sending the signal further into the brain. Another pathway is through nerves leading to the brain, whose electrical signals provide information about the body. One such nerve is the vagus nerve, the "wandering nerve" that sends sensory information from the body's internal organs up to the brainstem. Both communication paths give an almost beautiful effect: the corresponding substances that triggered the signal somewhere in the body now begin to be produced inside the brain. Inflammation is thus mirrored inside the brain, perhaps as a way of understanding the events taking place in other parts of the body. Direct communication in very simple creatures became well-developed long-distance communication in more complex organisms such as mammals and other species with a separate and protected brain. The same substances are more or less central to molluscs' and humans' sickness behavior. If, like me, you are also feeling that the boundary between the concepts *body* and *soul* are starting to fade, I can contribute to that sense with another example. The same immune cells that secrete inflammatory cytokines in a mollusc can also secrete stress hormones on their own. That is to say, a simple stress response can be performed by the mollusc's immune cell, even in the absence of a brain capable of coordinating a fight or flight response. No troublesome disciplinary boundaries there, right?

But back to humans, and to your brain that time you felt miserably ill. Inflammatory substances sent a signal to your brain, caused some inflammatory activity, and managed to adjust the systems that control your motivation and behavior. Voilà—your sense of illness. So the brain controls the body, but the body also controls the brain.

Benjamin L. Hart is an American biologist who, as professor emeritus of veterinary medicine, dedicates much of his time to writing books and papers on high-priority scientific topics such as elephant brain evolution, the perfect puppy, dog penis morphology, wild animals' use of herbal medicine, and how to diagnose dogs that try to get attention by faking medical problems. Earlier in his career, in 1988, he published an important scientific article that gained widespread attention. The title of the article was "Biological basis of the behavior of sick animals." Hart had compiled a great deal of research on how animals behave when they are sick, or more specifically, when they have an infection. But Hart brought forth something new: a coherent theory suggesting that the behavior change was not due primarily to the weakness that the disease caused. Rather, it was an evolutionarily developed strategy to strengthen the body's defense against the lethal threat posed by the infection. Hart argued that the behavioral changes were an important part of immune defence. The changes showed numerous signs of being adaptive, meaning that they were genetic adaptations to the prevailing environment that increased the chances of surviving and passing along the genes. Hart described the functions but could not at that time know how the immune system could regulate the brain.[2]

For an organism under threat, energy-saving changes can make the difference between life and death, as that energy can be used for fever production or the white blood cells' war against infectious agents. According to Hart, a number of observations supported this perspective. As I mentioned earlier, raising body temperature is costly for metabolism, which is why behaviors that reduce the loss of energy and heat are prioritized. Thus, the desire to eat, to move, and to socialize with others is reduced. Increased pain or sensitivity to pain reduces the desire to move. Reduced food intake reduces the amount of available iron, which is problematic for bacteria which use iron to reproduce. At the same time, the risk of exposure to predators or hostile species is reduced. Hart noted that sick animal behaviors are quite similar to those of people: "This picture of the lethargic, depressed, anorexic, and febrile individual is not specific to any particular animal species but is seen in humans and a variety of animals, and the behavioral signs are seen with a variety of systemic diseases as well as with some more localized infections."[3]

Behavior is regulated by motivation—reduced desire to eat, of course, reduces food intake. Behavior is influenced by motivation toward a goal: to increase the chance of being healthy. This is what is behind your subjective feeling on those days when an internal battle is taking place in your body. Hart's observation that sick animals curl up to stay warm and save energy makes me think about the somewhat slumped posture of sick (and depressed) people. Could the origin of this be a remnant of "curling up

---

[2] In the same year (but published the year after), Hart wrote another groundbreaking article that described how animals also keep healthy through avoidance. This research describes behaviors that complement the sickness response and is described in Chapter 5.

[3] Hart BL. Biological basis of the behavior of sick animals. Neuroscience and biobehavioral reviews. 1988;12(2): p 123.

animal" behavior? Or a signal to others that you are out of commission? We do not know the answer, but we can conclude that "with a lowered head" appears as a literary expression, and that sick or depressed people tend to be depicted in the arts with lowered heads and a slumped posture.

There is a further aspect of the sickness response that is familiar to many, but which has been difficult to measure. Together with a decreased interest in interacting with one's environment, is there also an increased interest in one's own body and what is happening in it? Here we return to the concept of interoception; that is, information about the state of our own body (described in Chapter 2). A common observation is that attention is turned inside, toward the body, when we are sick. Perhaps it is no surprise if we now have bodily symptoms that shout "hello!" to the brain? We feel pain, feverish, tired, downhearted, and ill at ease. You can view it as a passive mechanism: with increased interoceptive signalling in the form of pain and other unpleasantness, it is natural that attention is directed inward rather than outward. But there can also be an active mechanism that helps to direct attention to the body. We shall return to such possible mechanisms and body focus in Chapter 5, in relation to how we assess our general state of health. There are clear systems in the brain to direct attention—a function that determines the difference between life and death in the myriad of impressions bombarding the brain from both our outer and inner worlds. Although we know little about the mechanisms by which inflammation increases attention toward the body, there is some support to the claim that attentional flexibility decreases with stronger inflammatory activity.

The question then arises whether the phenomenon of directing more attention to the body when ill (to the extent it is true) is good or bad. Annoyingly, the correct answer is only that the question is wrong. As a survival mechanism, increased bodily attention is excellent in an acute phase. Or has been, at least. The impression that this response pattern is important is reinforced by the observation that the mechanisms of sickness behavior are quite similar and strongly preserved throughout the so-called animal kingdom. And it is also likely that there are negative consequences of directing extra attention to the body when the inflammation does not subside—when the obstacle to living an ordinary life becomes too great, and when we find it difficult to motivate ourselves to do things that require effort but which result in only delayed gratification.

Before antibiotics, when infections were a leading threat to survival, it was likely excellent, for a limited time, to focus on the body's internal drama and listen carefully to the body's condition. If nothing else, it helped to keep still, right? This is certainly also advantageous for shorter periods of time, even for our own bodies and brains which we move around with in today's society. But probably not for longer time periods. It is difficult to interact with others, to justify doing things that meet only our long-term needs, and to work and accomplish things if we do not distribute our attention in a balanced way. An increasing number of health conditions are linked to chronic low-grade inflammation, which can contribute to dysfunction that likely adds insult to injury for those affected. Depressive symptoms and fatigue can be associated with low-grade inflammation, which can be a partial explanation for long-term problems common to many health conditions.

As with the stress response, it is important that the sickness response is turned on quickly and turned off when no longer necessary. Proper regulation of the inflammation process is thus of great importance to our health, and in a wider behavioral and social perspective.

Making people sick

Substances used to induce inflammation and sickness in lab animals can also be administered to humans. Let me tell you about one of my own experiences. After a long period of preparation—and a lot of hard work from former graduate student Bianka Karshikoff who skilfully organized all the practical details—our research group was granted the go-ahead to give a so-called endotoxin to humans. As I described in Chapter 3, an endotoxin is a part of a bacteria that the immune system recognizes. If it is only presented with an endotoxin, the immune system responds as if an infection is imminent and will trigger an inflammatory response—a fake infection, so to speak.

We wanted to study brain function using an MR scanner during the inflammatory response, test pain functions by repeatedly "hurting" people, and examine behavior and subjective experiences. In short, we wanted to create a safe model for sickness in which a person could come to our lab, feel appropriately sick for a few hours, and then go home and continue life as usual, unlike people with chronic illness, whom we were hoping to better understand. Yes, people do this to themselves voluntarily, and we, of course, carefully followed all the ethical guidelines to ensure that our studies were conducted safely. Personally, I was incredibly eager to receive the endotoxin injection and experience the sickness response that I had been interested in for so many years.

During the pre-tests, I became a test subject in order to ascertain what dosage to use. Research studies on sepsis treatments used the same substance but at a much higher dose. Our area of interest was the feeling of illness that is often linked to chronic but mild activation of the inflammatory system, as opposed to something that would be relevant within a hospital's intensive care unit. But the question of dose still presented us with a dilemma: if we were going to start these complicated and expensive trials, we wanted to be sure that we would get a reliable effect, and this could only be ensured with a higher dose. However, we didn't want it to be too easy for the trial subjects (or leaders) to guess whether they had been given an endotoxin or a placebo, or for them to feel too sick to crawl into the MR scanner.

I was the worst test subject imaginable. An hour or so after the injection I started feeling poorly and became increasingly aware of a feeling of discomfort crawling through my body. I pictured the white blood cells identifying the characteristic molecular pattern of bacteria, a pattern known as "pathogen-associated," and setting in motion the production of cytokines. But despite my discomfort I was exhilarated. How wonderfully interesting to be given the opportunity to study the phenomenon from an inside perspective, in good company, and in a controlled environment! A feeling of general discomfort—which fascinated me, which I knew the cause of, and which I knew would abate in a few hours—was undoubtedly different from the symptoms that would make most people consider cancelling trips, or those that are part of a chronic illness. White lab coats surrounded me, all safety equipment was within reach, and an MR scanner measured my brain functions. What more could you ask of a regular day at the office? I hatched a thousand new research ideas and conversed manically with my colleagues. On the whole I was feeling pretty good. It was not until the pain sensitivity test that I started feeling properly sick, much to the delight of my colleagues.

One of the pain tests was conducted in the following way: a researcher pressed a pressure sensor against the trapezius muscle in my neck, first lightly, then gradually with more force. My task was to communicate when the pressure began to turn into pain. This is called a pain threshold, and the method of measuring it produces an objective value for pain, which is a subjective phenomenon. These thresholds are, not surprisingly, lower for people suffering from fibromyalgia and other conditions that cause chronic pain—for example, a lot less pressure is needed to induce pain in these patients. We suspected that, for a few hours, the inflammation induced by the endotoxin would make us more similar to people with pain disorders. When something is very painful, the brain subdues the experience of pain by triggering a pain-inhibiting reaction. This reaction does not seem to work as it should in patients with chronic pain and they appear to have less activity in an area of the frontal lobe that starts this important pain-inhibiting response. The response is tested by examining the pain threshold when applying pressure to a muscle while at the same time also doing something painful, like submerging the lower arm in ice water. The strong pain in the arm triggers a pain-inhibition response, which allows for harder pressure on the neck muscle before the pressure turns into pain. I assure you, having your arm submerged in ice-cold water really hurts, and I was now wishing I didn't have a body full of agitated white blood cells that had been conned into releasing inflammatory products, exacerbating the pain. One of my younger colleagues was exceptionally happy to see that I was now responding appropriately, and jovially reported that it was the first time she had seen somebody literally turn green! But I was still well enough to go into the brain scanner so that we could find out if it could detect any effects of the endotoxin and inflammation running rampant in my body. John Axelsson, a close colleague who also led these experiments, is a former heavyweight boxer; despite his physique, he was feeling much worse than I was (much to my delight). Nevertheless, he also managed to lie down in the brain scanner, so we deduced that the dosage was probably enough to suit our purpose: to study a relatively mild inflammatory reaction and its effects on the brain.

The fact that we can induce a temporary inflammatory reaction in experiments allows us to understand how the immune system affects both our physical and mental health. It can also help us understand how processes in the body affect how we feel in a more general sense. There are other methods in addition to endotoxin that are used to understand how inflammation affects how we feel, think, and behave.

Perhaps you have noticed how you or a child reacts after a vaccination? Some inoculated patients report feeling tired a few hours after a vaccination, and one can often observe how children become cranky after having been injected. These responses to routine vaccinations and those we have to endotoxin injections in the lab have a similar cause. They are connected to the body's inflammatory response to the "threat," in this case a vaccine, that it perceives. This is also why vaccination is studied in research similar to ours, in which test subjects are asked to complete different tasks or report how they feel whilst in an MR scanner a few hours after receiving a typhoid inoculation. Within a few hours, the vaccination gives rise to a mild but significant increase in inflammatory products that resembles the reaction to endotoxin. A more drastic model involves administering a *real* infection to people by injecting them with live microorganisms. Consider also *pyrotherapy*, once used to treat syphilis, in which the patient was given malaria, causing a fever that killed the syphilis bacteria, and was then saved from malaria with quinine.

By giving endotoxin to people and then studying how their brains and behavior are affected by this or by vaccinations, it has become clear from many research groups that the insula is activated during a sickness response. This fits nicely with the model of interoception I presented in Chapter 2. In our own research, we have observed that the anterior insula is activated more when painful pressure is put on a person's thumb if they have been given endotoxin rather than a placebo. We have also observed a weaker than normal activation of the pain-inhibiting area in the anterior cingulum. As we had expected, test subjects began to show more similarities to chronic pain patients both in terms of increased pain sensitivity and activation patterns in the brain. Following this kind of immune activation, the insula also appears to be more active while at rest (for example, when subjects are not exposed to pain or asked to complete tasks), and we have observed, in our experiments, a stronger connection between the anterior insula and the middle cingulum. Researchers studying the brain's reward system have seen changes there that further strengthen our overall understanding of sickness response after inflammatory impact on the brain—changes that make individuals more pain-sensitive, depressed, and tired and less motivated to participate in activities outside the home. Less sensitive to reward, and more sensitive to negative events, it seems like.

Inner threats and common symptoms

In many disease states, there are specific symptoms that give doctors important clues about what is happening in the body so that a correct diagnosis can be made. But the model of sickness described in this chapter is actually relevant even when you do not have an infection, that is, when you have not been invaded by microorganisms, and also applies to injuries and other health conditions that we will return to later. The model is therefore important in describing the way we and our bodies react when we are sick in a *general sense* and not only as a result of a specific disease state. We can therefore conceive of the sickness response as a generalized reaction to threats that we are exposed to at the micro level, a response that generally increases our odds of becoming healthy across conditions.

To get some perspective on this idea, let's rewind to 1923, to the time of the exceptionally creative physician and researcher Hans Selye. Selye was born in Vienna, Austria-Hungary, studied medicine in Prague, and eventually emigrated to Canada after working in the United States. Eager, cocky, and deeply knowledgeable about preclinical medicine, he one day participated in a "patient demonstration" where a professor of infectious diseases presented patients to the medical students. The aim was to learn to recognize typical signs of the infectious diseases the patients suffered from and make a correct diagnosis. Selye saw no specific signs that indicated which infection diagnosis was the right one. However, he saw a variety of symptoms that all of the patients seemed to be suffering from. They complained about diffuse pain and appetite problems, and many of them felt confused. Not only did they feel sick, they looked sick. These symptoms were clear, but ignored by the teacher, who instead enumerated a list of symptoms that would help in diagnosing the disease. Selye thought the specific signs of the disease were difficult to spot, and the professor acknowledged that they "happened to be absent" at that time. Selye then suggested to the professor that he be given access to a lab to do research. When asked what he planned to study, he replied, "the general syndrome of being sick," which was followed by ridicule. Along the same line, he was also known for asking stupid questions such as, "why do sick people look alike?" No wonder Selye returned to the classroom and to his successful studies. When he later made another attempt at research, he focused on the hormone system, taking extracts from various organs and injecting them into rodents. The changes he saw in some of their organs made him think that he had discovered a new hormone. He then conducted control experiments with other preparations, but each one produced similar changes. He noted that even untreated animals that happened to escape, and which he had to hunt down in the lab, showed similar changes.

Selye was close to giving up on the idea of research altogether when he thought of all the patients he saw who had similar symptoms despite having a variety of illnesses. What if this was the body's general response to threats? He started talking about "irritants" and "noxious agents" before eventually starting to adopt the (already sometimes used) term "stress." With support from his observations, he described how the immune system was affected by stress hormones, and how the main reaction was immune system stimulation. In the development of research on stress—a valid, important, and difficult concept—its connection to the general disease syndrome and to the patients who, according to Selye, even looked similar, was lost. But not forever.

Times have changed. Immunology has identified relevant signalling substances. These substances' dialogue with the nervous system has been described, and new brain imaging methods have given us access to the living human brain. Psychoneuroimmunology is rapidly spreading into a number of related research fields. The physiological bases for emotions, thoughts, and assessments are being mapped. Enter the subjective world and our complex feelings about health.

There are great similarities between what we call stress and the sickness response, a statement that will not surprise you if I have succeeded in describing the body's *general* systems for addressing threats. At the macro level, the threats can be about how to manage the risk of violence or how to cope with work, and the reorganization of imminent behaviors. At the micro level, there may be potentially deadly microorganisms that must be destroyed. Some of the terminology used in immunology seems to be inspired by the literature on threats, fear, and stress. For example, collective terms such as "danger-associated molecular patterns" are used for molecules that release responses similar to the bacterial stimuli we injected into research volunteers and ourselves. Administration of bacterial molecules is then not about precise infectious agents, but about the *commonalities* across many infectious agents, and which give rise to generalized changes in the body—changes that, in many cases, have successfully increased survival (that is, "things to watch out for"). And similar to external threats, behavior is part of the successful strategy for dealing with internal threats.

If different types of threats activate a set of relatively similar responses in order to increase the chance of survival, we should, as Selye envisioned, see symptoms that are relatively similar across different types of illnesses—and this has proven to be the case. Many of the symptoms that drive people to healthcare providers are related to pain, fatigue, depression, appetite changes, and sleep, and are sometimes called transdiagnostic. Such symptoms represent a large part of the suffering during illness, and are not always directly linked to a specific disease mechanism, but rather to a general survival strategy triggered in humans and animals when confronting a threat. Understanding the mechanisms behind such general symptoms is therefore important.

Threats in the social world

The human brain is adapted to a social life. This enables us to take care of our offspring for a long time, live together for shorter or longer periods, and function in large groups. The ability of an individual to pass on their genes is strongly influenced by their place in the group, and in this context, interpersonal violence is an obvious danger. Social threats are therefore highly relevant, and consequently, both the hormone system and the immune system are affected when faced with social challenges. Being evaluated by others is viewed by most people as stressful, and this fact is often used in a model for studying stress. During such an experiment, the subject may perform a speech task and at the same a demanding arithmetical calculation. The possibility that one's performance may be negatively evaluated, especially if the subject does not have control over the situation, boosts the hormones cortisol, adrenaline, and norepinephrine. In addition, genes are activated to produce inflammatory cytokines. If there is no audience, the effect is less, even if the subject perceives the situation and task as equally challenging, difficult to control, and tricky. If we study the relationship between social factors, the immune system, and the health of people in society (rather than that of individuals), our understanding of the importance of social relationships is strengthened. For example, there are strong relationships between socioeconomic status (not only objective but also "experienced") and various aspects of health. Loneliness has been linked to gene expression related to the increase in so-called pro-inflammatory substances and to the down-regulation of anti-inflammatory substances (for example, cytokines that counteract inflammatory processes). Similar to perceived socioeconomic status, *perceived* loneliness is a risk factor for morbidity and mortality, regardless of the objective level of social isolation and health behaviors. One's subjective experience once again proves to be important for key measures of health and well-being.

It is clear that the inflammatory system can be activated (or prepared for activity through a phenomenon called *priming*) by many factors that are not directly linked to infection. It is logical that threats, such as losing status in a dominance hierarchy, activate these systems in anticipation of coming consequences. From the perspective of social threats, it is reasonable to assume that they pose an increased risk of external threats, such as interpersonal violence along with subsequent tissue damage and exposure to infectious agents, which in the next phase may pose an internal health threat. It is therefore reasonable that behavior is used both to increase the chance of recovery from illness (through sickness behavior) and to reduce the risk of becoming ill (through avoidance behavior). And because we live in a highly social world, your perception of the outside world is of great interest to your inner bodily processes.

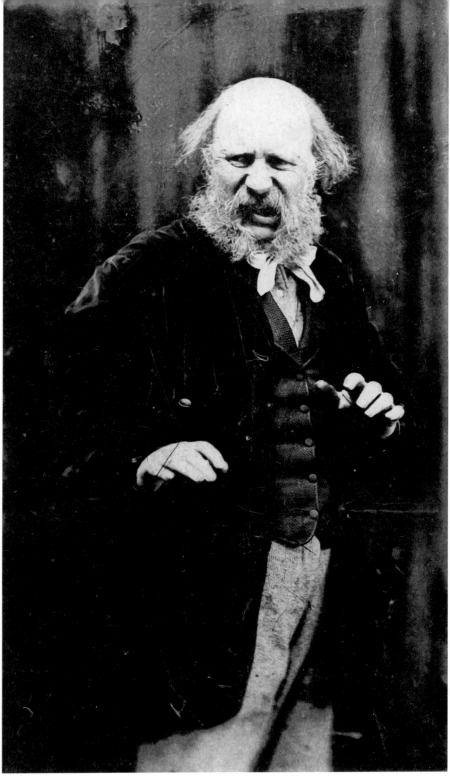

An expression of disgust

5

DISGUST AND PREJUDICE IN DISEASE DEFENSE

The sickness response is a reactive part of illness, so that the chance of recovery increases thanks to the immune system's communication with the brain and the altered behavior that follows. But if we think about how crucial infection defense is for all kinds of animals, it is worth reflecting on the role of behavior in building a total defense system against infection.

With an acidic and inhospitable environment in the skin and mucous membranes, we have barriers that defend the borders and make invasion more difficult. If it does happen, we still have white blood cells that, like soldiers, can be prepared for action when a threat is approaching, and activated to use their arsenal of weapons when the time comes. But to build a total defense system, we also need a security policy to reduce the risk of conflict and invasion. A defense system should therefore include proactive elements so that a person behaves in a way that reduces their risk of becoming ill. Such features would be particularly relevant when the risk of infection is high. One consequence of this reasoning is that a person should be able to feel or assume that another person may be ill. Another consequence is that this suspicion should be greater when the general threat level is higher. Continuing down this path, that subjective threat perception could even cause one's own defense mechanisms within the body to remain on alert. Although research on behaviors that have evolved to *avoid* infection is still in its infancy, it is clear that it constitutes a completely natural and unique entity, along with its reactive cousin, the sickness response. With this knowledge, the history of the brain and immune system

The Inflamed Feeling. Mats Lekander, Oxford University Press. © Mats Lekander 2022.
DOI: 10.1093/oso/9780198863441.003.0005

clearly becomes even more remarkable. Let's think about whether your attitude toward other people, who you want to avoid, or even your political values, could be related to disease risk.

Here I present the remarkable story of how illness risk is related to norms, taboos, xenophobia, and our tendency to like good-looking people. It is not a beautiful story, but fascinating.

Disease avoidance

The influence of stress and conditioning on the immune system were early cornerstones in the field of psychoneuroimmunology. Following the discovery of communication mechanisms between the nervous and immune systems, a solid foundation could be laid. Slowly, the area evolved from a collection of diffuse opinions (often expressed as, "I think that emotions may affect one's ability to stay healthy") to one that could be described and studied using standard accepted scientific methodology—from beliefs based on introspection and values to knowledge based on established methods. Test tubes, microscopes, brain imaging, reliable measurement of subjective experiences using statistics and scrutiny—far from "new age" and "pseudoscience"[1]—are tools that can be found in nearly any medical science toolbox and, for some time too, in this research field also. But still, it is mind-boggling that a feeling, if it is significant and persistent, in some sense can be perceived by the white blood cells and affect their search for invaders or damaged cells.

Early on, studies on sickness responses and the immune system's control of the brain began to appear within psychoneuroimmunology. These

---

[1] The scientifically defined mechanisms in psychoneuroimmunology have been heavily borrowed by pseudoscientific practitioners who have sought scientific credibility in order to sell treatments, products, and beliefs. My view, however, is that, despite its challenging subjects, psychoneuroimmunology has succeeded quite well in keeping non-scientific methods and practitioners at bay. The subject's flagship journal *Brain, Behavior, and Immunity* has gradually earned a place among top-tier scientific journals in neuroscience and immunology.

areas have continued to increase over the last decade or two, and have now more formally, under the name immunopsychiatry, entered psychiatry research. But a new wave of research is now emerging, with the aim of understanding the role behavior plays in the "security policy" of the total immunological defense system.

I am now referring to the avoidance of illness and to what is sometimes called a behavioral immune system (which should also include the sickness response not to be an obvious misnomer) or even a social immune system. Fascinating data indicates how we actively avoid infection, and that this tendency affects behaviors that we believe are based on completely different motivations than illness prevention. With this system, infectious agents can be managed, not only through the aggressive activities of our white blood cells, but also by reducing the probability that we are at risk from the start. Since infectious agents are not visible to the naked eye, a system has been developed that, through superficial signs, values, and social behavior, keeps us away from possible sources of infection. These ideas are summarized in an overall theory of how we can avoid illness and how this affects our behavior.

Like other evolution-based theories,[2] it has a distinctive advantage and an equally distinctive disadvantage. The advantage is that it provides meaning; it summarizes and explains a large amount of data and observations that are otherwise unrelated. The power of explanation is enormous. A large number of predictions can be made that can then be tested—is the reality we study consistent with the predictions we can make from this evolutionary perspective? The downside is that the theory is difficult to test experimentally; we can only gather indirect support for it, and that means that evolutionarily inspired theories can be wild, with human imagination its strongest limiting factor. However, combined support for the evolutionary theory of genetic mutations, selection and

---

[2] A theory is something that summarizes data to explain phenomena in a systematic way. It differs from how the term is sometimes used in daily speech, where it represents more of an assumption, which in scientific language is called a hypothesis.

spread of genes that increase survival, and the important role of behavior in this area is extremely strong.

Okay, enough caveats. On to the world of behaviors that seems to have been created to address one of the greatest challenges—perhaps the greatest—to the human genome: the threat from parasitic microorganisms that want to infect you and your loved ones and take advantage of the ideal environment for reproduction that the human interior offers. We shall consider a number of phenomena that we all know about and often have experience with, keeping the theory of disease avoidance in the back of our heads. Or, if I may suggest, in the front of our heads—a neuroanatomically more reasonable place for working memory.

Behaviors that decrease the risk of disease

As a first example, we will start at the beginning of life and ask why nausea is so common in expectant mothers at the beginning of pregnancy. It is easy to understand that nutritional exactitude is important for the protection of both the fetus and the mother, and that nausea contributes to the general caution of the mother during the most sensitive period of embryonic development. At the same time, the immune cells' activity is important in managing the defense against microorganisms that enter the body, while the risk of expelling the fetus must at the same time be minimized. After all, it is made up of new and semi-foreign cells rapidly growing inside the mother's body and could be mistaken as dangerous. What could be more appropriate than being assisted by behavior so that the relative suppression of the immune cells' activity, necessary at the beginning of pregnancy, does not increase the risk of the mother and child becoming infected? Key players in the immune system, the white blood cells, decrease their activity during this period, but the external defense system of behavior is strengthened. Nausea guides expectant mothers toward food with a low risk of causing infection, because it is now easier to feel disgust. During the first months of pregnancy we can see that mothers are closer to the disgust emotion. These emotional responses serve to reduce the risk of poisoning and infection. Disgust is also part of how we react to our own or others' moral transgressions, which can leave "a bad taste in your mouth." It is likely that because toxic and contagious substances are invisible, rules and taboos help prevent us from doing things that, despite deficient evidence, may be dangerous to us. A reaction that began by protecting the mouth against infectious agents has developed to contribute both to the protection of the body generally as well as to social order and morality.

Therefore it could be that, during pregnancy, the tendency toward more nausea and disgust is manifested in judgments and opinions related to other people, and how one views behavior that defies social boundaries or taboos. Accordingly, there are studies that show that mothers' general values change during pregnancy so that their attitudes toward strangers become more negative and cautious. The basic tendency people have toward ethnocentrism (judging other cultures based on one's own group values and norms) is reinforced in pregnant women at a time when they particularly need to protect the fetus, so that they value their own group even more than usual. A classic study by Navarrete and colleagues from 2007 showed how attitudes towards one's own group changed during pregnancy, with significantly higher ethnocentrism during the first infection-sensitive trimester of pregnancy, then decreasing. Interestingly, the change in ethnocentrism was almost parallel with the change in nausea: first an increase and then a decrease. The occurrence of nausea and altered values in pregnancy is one of many phenomena that advocate for, but do not prove, the theory that behavior is used as one component of a total defense against infection. The benefit is obvious: the risk of infection is great during the sensitive time when organs are formed because the embryo can be damaged and white blood cells can reject the fetus during excessive activity. Enter behavior.

What we think of as the immune system in everyday language (white blood cells and other protective features like the mucous membrane's physical barrier and inhospitable environment) comprises mechanisms that respond to *microscopic clues* about infectious agents that have entered the body. A behavioral part of the immune defense helps provide *perceptual clues* about the risk of being exposed to those agents. But it is only inside the body that small structures such as bacteria or viruses can be detected. But with the help of eyes and ears we can perceive larger threats. Added to this are the chemical sensory reactions: smell and taste. And in addition, thoughts and emotions contribute additional building blocks to the total immunological defense system needed to thrive and survive.

Since infectious agents such as bacteria and viruses are dangerous, but too small to be directly observed outside the body, humans also respond to a number of very general clues about what *could* occur in the environment. It can be people who seem sick, food that is unfamiliar or seems old, or even people who do not belong to what we regard as "our group." It may be, for example, individuals from foreign cultures. When the threat is great, the cost of a false positive reaction (responding to a false alarm) is low, while the cost of a false negative reaction (not detecting and therefore failing to respond to a true risk) can be devastating: infection or poisoning that weakens or even kills. Therefore, from an evolutionary perspective, excessive suspicion can be beneficial, especially in times of increased threat (such as pregnancy or danger).

Suspicion then falls upon our fellow human beings who *could* be sick or who could possibly carry a variety of foreign microorganisms. Individuals who, on flimsy and unfair grounds, can be assumed to belong to groups other than our own, could pose a risk of carrying an organism that could kill us, or if not, still diminish the opportunity to pass on our genes.

Even our "traditional" immune system often errs on the side of caution and can respond to a variety of benign stimuli that could potentially be harmful. One of many examples of excessive sensitivity is allergy, when harmless pollen triggers a response in white blood cells. Allergy has a striking resemblance to phobias in the sense that the innate protection system is dysregulated and activated to such an extent that it transitions into a disease state. In immunology, this is a classic problem: understanding how cells are trained to recognize but not respond to bodily substances. White blood cells develop a tolerance to these substances in a very refined way, but the boundary between self and non-self, and between the dangerous and harmless, is so complicated that the process often goes awry. In autoimmune diseases, the self/non-self trade-off fails, resulting in an attack on our bodily structures by our own protective system.

Taken together, this indicates that the management of different types of threats represents a difficult balancing act for living organisms. How much activity is sufficient, and how should the enemy be identified? Behavior is a key element in managing threats and is largely involved in the balance between cost (how much energy to spend on defense) and benefit (how much an organism can gain by scaling up or disarming a given threat). Because the systems are so advanced and need to be calibrated to adapt to the prevailing needs of our modern world, the development and adjustment of these systems takes place over a long period of time, starting before birth and proceeding for a long time thereafter. Therefore, the immediate environment we are exposed to throughout our lives contributes to how our bodies calibrate our level of sensitivity to various health risks. In other words, genes and environment interact constantly. In addition, everything is affected by our behavior, which affects our health, and our health ultimately affects what we do and how we feel.

How your endeavor to stay healthy affects your values

Since infectious agents such as viruses or bacteria can be dangerous but not visible to the naked eye, protection to becoming exposed to these substances is largely governed by norms, values, and agreements. We respond with disgust to food that looks old, smells rancid, or reminds us of something unpleasant, and the function of this emotion is to make us spit out what we ingest or completely avoid something (or someone). As I described earlier, we react with this basic emotional system even to violations of moral codes or taboos. If you believe that a certain type of sexual contact is wrong, you react with disgust when you think about it. If you have the culturally conditioned view that you should not eat dogs, shell food, cow, or perhaps pig, your reaction is the same—the thought of crossing that boundary raises feelings of distaste and disgust, perhaps even a slight sense of nausea. When you experience disgust for repulsive food, you pull up your lips and wrinkle your nose. The same muscles are activated by looking at others who behave in a selfish and morally dubious manner. Using this same reasoning, we also approach the subject of attitudes and prejudices toward people who we perceive as not belonging to our own group. For our ancestors, this was a way of avoiding not only the risk of violence, but also the risk of being infected with harmful agents. These infectious substances can be completely harmless to the foreign person, but deadly dangerous if the substances are not already a natural part of their lives.

Research has clarified some unpleasant phenomena that show how close we are to ill-founded conclusions and prejudices about other people, and that these reactions are actually biologically programmed. The tendencies are not motivated or true just because evolution has contributed to them. Descriptions of how things are, like other scientific conclusions that describe and explain the world, carry no value and cannot in themselves be accurate measures of whether things are good or bad. Few things are entirely "natural," but are shaped by the current environment and its cultural factors. But by looking at genetically predisposed phenomena, we can better understand some inherent tendencies to all kinds of folly. Seen from an evolutionary perspective—the possibility of passing on genes during the course of development—they become understandable. As for fear, there are a number of studies that show that we can more easily learn fear linked to the faces of people with a different skin color than our own, and that this fear is more difficult to extinguish. The phenomenon is similar to what one sees when learning and extinguishing the fear of snakes and spiders; fear of these animals is easier to learn, and harder to eliminate, than for other animals or objects. This elevated tendency seems to be genetically ingrained and appears to be the reason why spider and worm phobia are so common, despite the fact that so many other things are more dangerous to modern man. One possible explanation is that genetically ingrained tendencies toward prejudice could have protected us from the risk of infection and other threats.

Our tendency to favor people who seem to belong to our "in-group" is reflected in brain activity when we see others being exposed to discomfort or pain. We react more strongly in brain areas related to compassion and empathy when we look at pictures or films of people of our own ethnicity who are exposed to pain. But this tendency is not just about ethnic origin as a sign of group affiliation; it can also be seen if we have more cultural and unstable reasons to believe that the person belongs to our own group. It can apply to something as simple as what football team the person seems to support, or that the person belongs to a group with a different tee-shirt color than the one we ourselves were assigned to wear during an experiment. We and them, from a biologically ingrained perspective, one might say. During experiments in which a supporter of an opposing football team is exposed to pain, not only is there reduced activity in the systems involved in compassion, but there is also increased activity in the brain's reward system. How typical of the human brain, I am tempted to think, before realizing that I am even more surprised that prejudice as an emotional reaction is at all possible to study through brain imaging technology.

Biologically predisposed tendencies can thus contribute to negative attitudes and prejudices, and the tendency to learn to fear foreign faces from ethnicities different than our own may have been a way to reduce the risk of being exposed to violence (the phenomenon is, by the way, strongest in regards to fear of male faces). But couldn't fear of the new, not least of other individuals, be related to disease avoidance, which over the course of evolution posed at least as great a threat to survival as violence? We should therefore be able to predict geographical variation in both degrees of fear of foreign individuals and degrees of openness to violations of norms and taboos in a manner—just as the threat of parasites varies greatly between different geographical areas. This would make sense from an infection perspective. And shouldn't we also be able to do experiments in which we trigger a fear of illness, and in this way increase an individual's sensitivity to norm violations and negative attitudes towards foreigners?

If we study geographical differences in the occurrence of parasites, we can see how values and attitudes towards foreigners also change. The term *parasite* here includes so-called microparasites, such as viruses or bacteria. A higher presence of parasites and worse health are generally associated with less openness, more conservative values, a higher degree of religiosity, and stronger xenophobia. Neophobia (fear of the new) is a good summary word for these trends. This may be due to numerous things apart from the risk of illness influencing behavior in a conservative direction. We do not know what causes what.

Countries in which the parasite threat is higher and that have a higher burden of infections are generally controlled by more authoritarian regimes. There is also a connection to being somewhat more religious, more collectivistic, and less open to experiences. Such differences also apply when comparing different regions within a country, such as different regions of the United States. There are also signs that individuals who feel more distaste for potential infectious agents and who are more aware of general infection risk have more conservative views. Therefore, similar to what has been shown about tendencies toward ethnocentricity when exposed to disease threats, it appears that values and attitudes are influenced by anti-parasite strategies that are more or less activated at the individual or group level.

If you perform experiments in which you raise the topic of illness, or show pictures of sick people, you can demonstrate how negative views toward other people increase temporarily. If we assume that we have a general tendency to avoid infection (and of course other threats) by being on our guard against individuals or groups we do not know, it is obvious that the built-in tendency to believe more in members of our own group is further strengthened as the threat level increases. It is also logical that the tendency will weaken as the threat level decreases. A loud noise puts us in a state of readiness and startles us if heard in an unsafe part of a city, while the same sound in our own home hardly makes us react at all. The sense of being in our own home is a safety signal to us, which supresses the nervous system's response to an unexpected noise, while the situation is different in dodgy neighborhoods. As described in Chapter 4, this phenomenon is called functional flexibility, where the strength of a general and genetically predisposed response pattern like this is modified and adapted to the context. This also applies to the avoidance of illness.[3]

Threats of illness and infection increase our tendency to be more cautious or even afraid of people of other origins. Navarrete and Fessler put it like this in 2006: "Since networks of alliances are the only health insurance policy available in small-scale societies, it follows that, when the likelihood of illness increases, individuals should be motivated to ensure both that their premiums are paid and that their coverage is extensive."

Fear of illness therefore triggers avoidance behaviors and seems to affect social contact patterns among people. There is no doubt that such reaction patterns are profoundly unfair and prejudicial in nature, as this entails that individuals are judged on the basis of group affiliation or superficial factors. They contribute to social injustice and cruelty when members of ethnic groups other than the dominant one are objectified, perhaps likened to infectious animals or regarded as unclean. We and them again, with a genetically ingrained tendency toward prejudice that we should be aware of. Historically, there have been many examples of how ethnic groups that are not our own have been described as animals associated with the transmission of disease, such as cockroaches, rats, and parasites, or as unhealthy, unclean, or "polluted." People who perceive themselves as susceptible to illness and those who feel easily disgusted display more negative attitudes toward people outside of their own group.

As I previously mentioned, more direct support for the link between disease defense and attitudes toward others comes from studies in which the perceived disease threat was manipulated during experiments.

---

[3] Navarrete CD, Fessler DMT. Disease avoidance and ethnocentrism: The effects of disease vulnerability and disgust sensitivity on intergroup attitudes. *Evol Hum Behav*. 2006;27(4):270–82.

Subjects who were exposed to pictures showing how easily bacteria and viruses can be transmitted in everyday life showed less positive attitudes toward immigrants they perceived as foreign compared to people who saw a series of pictures showing how easily accidents can happen. Another experiment showed that people who read a history of swine flu showed less prejudice against foreign groups if they were already vaccinated against swine flu, and especially if they perceived the vaccination as effective. Even washing their hands with a cleansing napkin reduced the connection between the threat of illness and prejudicially biased attitudes.

Thinking back on the comparisons between information coming from the inner and the outer worlds, and how they are processed in the body and the brain, we may now see another parallel between these two systems. This time, when sensitivity to a threat is too great, and an innate response pattern is dysregulated and overactivated, it becomes a handicap. It can even form the basis for severely handicapping psychiatric disorders.

At a conference I organized, the American scientist Mike Davis presented a case showing how the innate tendency to respond to a sudden noise (an orientation response) can cause problems if not properly regulated and inhibited when appropriate. A Vietnam veteran who suffered from post-traumatic stress disorder (PTSD) came out of the church at his wedding when a car suddenly backfired. The wedding guests stopped and simply noticed what had happened—they were in a safe environment where no dangers were expected, nothing more. The groom, on the other hand, had thrown himself straight down into a dirty ditch. A wedding, 25 years after Vietnam, at home in the United States, wearing a white tuxedo instead of military attire—signals of safety were everywhere, but the signals' message about a safe context was not enough to inhibit a response that had been sensitized and overly reactive for many years. Here we see a response to an *external* signal whose basis is innate—to respond to a loud and unexpected sound—but which, for the war veteran, cannot be inhibited by the context. It scared him to such a great extent that the behavioral response, no matter how inappropriate, could not be stopped in time.

If we again focus on internal threats and dangers, we see a phenomenon that fits like a glove with this book's theme on subjective health factors—namely, hypochondriasis. This disorder is common among people seeking medical care, and one characteristic is that the fear of illness is not significantly affected by medical examinations that prove an absence of disease, but lives its own life. A better term that means roughly the same thing as hypochondriasis[4] is *health anxiety*. It says a lot about the core of the problem: bodily sensations are interpreted in a way that make you think you are suffering from a serious illness. However, the fear can be there without bodily symptoms and can be related to the fear of becoming sick. Connected to health anxiety is the fear that other people are sick and that you will become sick if you get too close to them. This is not so surprising, and can be difficult for the patient's social life. This brings us back to our tendency to want to avoid infection.

With health anxiety, the natural tendency to limit contact with potentially contagious people, and the equally natural tendency to take bodily symptoms seriously, overreact and are thus misaligned. The fear of the threat we cannot see, but merely presume based on diffuse bodily signals, is unreasonably strong. For people with health anxiety, the fear cannot be controlled by safety signals alone. Healthcare providers' repeated assurances that one is healthy does not help. These individuals are major healthcare consumers. Regardless of the suffering that health anxiety causes, the difference between subjective and objective health among these individuals is fascinating and compels me, as if it were needed, to provide a long defense of subjectively perceived health in Chapter 6. But first, the reasoning behind how we avoid illness, and what it has to do with our values, norms, and behaviors.

---

[4] The Greek origin of the word hypochondriasis has to do with the part of the abdomen that lies under the cartilage of the breastbone. It was thought that evaporations from the abdomen up to the chest and the head gave rise to discomfort and confusion. Until the beginning of the nineteenth century, hypochondriasis was tantamount to melancholy.

How can we know when others are sick?

I have discussed how prejudices, norms, values, and assumptions about increased risk of infection can provide a basis for influencing our behaviors. But can we actually perceive when others are sick? If we are to avoid one of the historically greatest threats to survival—infection—it must be useful to have other concrete and accurate clues beyond group affiliation. Such clues can then trigger avoidance behaviors and thereby reduce the risk of infection.

We know from experiments that animals' social relationships and behaviors are severely affected when they are ill, which I briefly discussed in Chapter 4. An important and somewhat less understood aspect of this is how animals' behavior is affected when they can detect illness in another animal. After all, avoiding illness has a different meaning if it is based not only on guesswork, but on whether tangible or even direct signs of illness can be perceived. From studies with animals, we know that they can have such an ability, and new research suggests that the same thing actually applies to humans.

Animals such as dogs and rodents have a well-developed sense of smell that can be utilized to detect danger, and they can use it to recognize physiological changes in others. Dogs seem able to be trained to recognize different types of tumors in humans via exhalation, urine, and tissue samples. If a tumor can be detected before it causes symptoms, treatment can be initiated earlier and important time saved. Some dogs are sold as diabetes alert dogs, and there is some, albeit mixed, evidence that they can detect too low or too high blood sugar levels and prompt owners to take action.

One may ask how specific an odor change is. Would it be evolutionarily advantageous to recognize the smell of inflammation? Can inflammations with different causes be distinguished, and would this be useful information? An inflammatory activation is, to a certain extent, a general response to many different types of infectious agents. But at the same time, inflammatory reactions also occur in response to events that do not involve infection, such as wounds, allergies, or autoimmune diseases. Researchers in the United States have shown that mice have some ability to distinguish different types of early inflammatory responses in other mice by smelling their urine. Not surprisingly, the detection of infection in other mice via the sense of smell is usually accompanied by avoidance of that individual, which can be presumed to be a way of avoiding infection. Although the animals, at least in some cases, can differentiate between different types of early inflammatory reactions, one can assume that the responses are similar, so that the recognition of inflammation (regardless of the risk of infection) increases the likelihood of avoidance behavior.

Let's return to dogs. There is another example related to the identification of highly contagious infections. Rapid identification of infectious diseases is important to prevent transmission, but identification through cell cultures takes time. In its Christmas editions, the *British Medical Journal* usually publishes quirky research articles, described as "light-hearted but rigorous." For Christmas 2012, they published an article about Cliff, an adorable two-year-old beagle. Cliff worked extra in Dutch hospitals, to identify *Clostridium difficile* infections. The bacterium is common, highly contagious, and can spread quickly in hospitals so that entire departments may need to be shut down. Early detection can thus make a big difference. Enter Cliff. After a training period, he either walked around among patients, where one in ten was infected with Clostridium, or directly smelled stool samples. If Cliff discovered the bacterium, he marked by sitting or lying down. Cliff identified 25 out of 30 infected patients just by walking around among them—not bad at all. But when it came to stool samples, the result was sensational: both sensitivity (the ability to detect a true infected sample) and specificity (not responding to a non-infected sample) were 100 percent! This means that Cliff was right every time he smelled a stool sample, accurately reporting if the bacterium was present or not.

But what about people? Here we are reminded of clinical medicine and how certain diseases are considered to be linked to particular smells. The scent of *scrofula*, a disease that can be caused by tubercle bacteria, has been described as stale beer; typhoid fever as freshly baked bread; and yellow fever as a butcher's shop. Cholera has been associated with a sweetish odor, and some tumor diseases with a rotting quality. Diabetes is perhaps the best-known example. When fatty acids are used as an energy source instead of glucose, acetone is one of the byproducts. This results in a fruity scent from urine and breath. Now you are surely wondering if it is not time for an "even the ancient Greeks" example, and how right you are. Hippocrates himself wrote about the scent of diseases and believed that smells from bodily fluids, like other impressions obtained through the doctor's sensory systems, could be helpful in diagnostics, and to some extent he was proven correct. Inspired by the possibility of recognizing diseases through the sense of smell, the development of "electronic noses" (sensors for various chemical substances connected to a computer) is underway, which can have broad applications.

The examples here apply to diseases that for some time have left their mark on affected individuals' physiological systems, and can certainly be useful in recognizing the same conditions in others. But from an evolutionary perspective, it would be even better if you could recognize infections at an early stage, when risk for contagion may be greatest. This brings us back to the inflammatory response, which starts very quickly after a contaminant enters a living organism. Would a person even be able to handle such a task? Humans' sense of smell may not be as powerful as that of many animals, and we are used to seeing ourselves as creatures that cannot use our sense of smell in any refined ways. But this can actually be called into question, and the sense of smell can in many cases be better in human beings than we think. The fact that we may be better than sensitive analytical instruments at detecting fragrances may say more about the instruments than about us, but what about people having lower detection thresholds than other primates when smelling some substances? Okay, but aren't those primates still pretty close to humans? Sure, but another fact is that we can beat both dogs and rats in detecting some specific types of chemical compounds.

This type of reasoning, and the great survival value that detecting early disease processes in others should present, made our research team decide to test whether humans can perceive the scent of inflammation. In the endotoxin experiments I described earlier, we had an opportunity, under the leadership of olfaction researcher Mats J. Olsson, to investigate this issue. When the subjects were injected with endotoxin or placebo and then participated in various tests, they were required to wear a tight tee-shirt and were not allowed to use deodorant. After four hours, each subject had to take off their tee-shirts, and the armpit regions were cut out and saved. At a later date, 40 other subjects were allowed to smell the samples stored in plastic bottles. By squeezing the bottles, they received a small puff of "healthy" or "sick" body odor. They then rated the samples for intensity, pleasantness, and health. The differences were not large, but statistically very clear: the "inflamed" scent samples were perceived as more intense, less pleasant, and less healthy. Next, we investigated whether we could observe these same effects again, through a new experiment (as one swallow doesn't make a summer). For this we also collected urine for use in a smell test, and tested people's abilities in the same way as (other) animals have previously been tested (although in my experience, we do not usually sniff one another each day). Some support has been presented that people smell more on their hands after shaking hands with another person. So what about the experiment with urine? Well, some evidence was in fact shown for a dissimilar smell in the "sick" versus "healthy" condition. Human capacity and use of the olfactory system may well surpass our preconceived ideas.

Given that the sense of smell is a chemical sensory system, it may work extra well in detecting diseases that can then affect behavior. The sense of smell is usually described as something that is not strongly linked to language, but that instead interprets a stimulus as either "good" or "bad," to thereby guide behavior. In order to describe the taste of wine, so-called descriptors have been established to better access tasting experiences that are otherwise difficult to articulate. So in our next study, our research team should perhaps ask people to describe the scent of disease in terms of "animal fur," "pencil shavings," "freshly cut garden," or "liquid Viagra."

What about other sensory systems? Can you see, hear, feel, or taste the health of others? Hippocrates described not only smelling patients, but also studying their appearance, touching them, listening to their chests, and even tasting their urine (see Figure 5.1). He advocated using all of the senses when observing patients so that the correct diagnoses could be

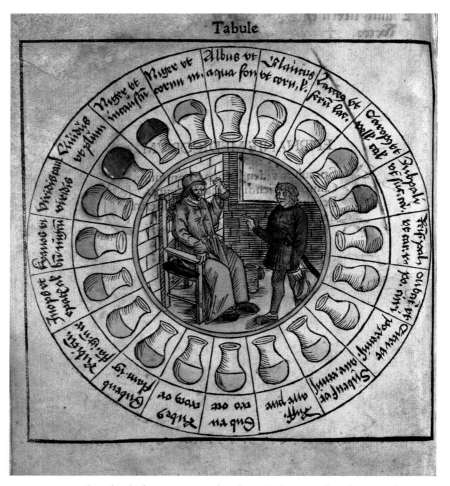

FIGURE 5.1 The wheel of urine was used in the early history of medicine to diagnose diseases based on the smell, taste, and color of the patient's urine.

Reproduced from Epiphanie medicorum. Speculum videndi urinas hominum. Clavis aperiendi portas pulsuum. Berillus discernendi causas et differentias febrium. [Ulrich Pinder]. Wellcome Collection. Attribution 4.0 International (CC BY 4.0)

made. Can we demonstrate, through experimental research, that we can recognize illness through these other senses? Taste is so closely related to odor that we will skip that one. In terms of vision, we have some knowledge about what people view as healthy, and the assessment of others' health, as reflected in their appearance, seems to be very important to us. There is a well-known relationship between attractiveness and health, so what we perceive as attractive in general is also a cue of good health. Likewise, attractiveness is considered to be a good hint of future health, that is, resistance to disease. In regions of the world where parasites are more common, the attractiveness of a partner is judged to be more important than in regions with lower parasite threats. This difference was also found to apply to regions in the United States. In parasite-dense regions, face symmetry is more important, as are expressions of female hormones (estrogen) in the face of a woman and male hormones (testosterone) in the face of a man. All this has been proposed to reflect a connection between different types of superficial cues of good health in relation to how great this need is with a partner and to the level of risk.

Surely these relationships could simply be expressions of culture that happen to coincide with the threat of parasites, without any causal relationships? Perfectly reasonable. But if you expose women and men in an experimental setting to images with a disease theme (suggesting a threat of illness), their preference for symmetry and hormonal markers in the faces of potential partners increases. This and similar examples indirectly support the idea of a connection between level of contagious disease threat and preferences for certain facial features. In summary, we generally seem to find that signs suggesting good health are attractive, but that circumstances also affect the extent to which this plays a role.

The Scottish professor David Perrett conducts research on facial color and health. I remember one of his surprising lectures particularly well; during his talk, he wore dramatic green and orange clothes, and his hair was beautifully colored to match the right and left sides of his outfit. Appropriately, Perrett has shown in his research that we perceive faces that contain more red and yellow tones as being generally healthier. This has an interesting parallel in the animal world, where the same colors act as cues of health and guides to attractive partner choices. For example, some birds with less bright colors on the beaks have weaker immune systems, and experiments with blackbirds have shown that their beaks fade if they become ill. The colors we have in our face, for example, are influenced by our lifestyle and will be stronger if we eat more fruit and vegetables. These changes in nuance depend on carotenoids—a group of yellow, red, and orange pigments with antioxidant properties.

Together with David Perrett, we have analyzed color changes in people with inflammation (who have received endotoxin) using an objective method (a so-called photo spectrometer), and have observed that the face loses some of its "redness" and becomes paler. When research volunteers who were not told about the endotoxin experiment were shown photos of the subjects' faces, they responded that those who received endotoxin looked sicker and more tired than those who received the placebo and could to some degree detect sickness from facial photos alone. But what cues were they most influenced by? It turns out that redder eyes and drooping eyelids are important, but also skin paleness and downturned corners of the mouth. Interestingly, the lips in particular were perceived as looking paler after immunostimulation, reminding me of the paler beaks displayed by blackbirds in similar experiments.

There is another feature of the visual system that is extremely sensitive and that could be used to detect cues of health conditions in others— namely, the analysis of motion. Motion is analyzed in several regions of the brain involved in vision, and motion that can be interpreted as coming from a living organism draws special attention. This is called *biological* motion and is important if we want to use the information to identify the source of the movement (what or who we see), or even say something about the internal state of the source in question. And we can. A particular part of the brain in the temporal lobe has proven to be particularly involved in understanding biological movement; not surprisingly, we use this area when reading lips.

The Swedish psychologist Gunnar Johansson showed early on how much information we can get from very limited movement information. He put small light sources on selected places on people's bodies and filmed them while they performed various tasks in the dark. When the people stood still, the bright spots provided absolutely no information to the viewer. But as soon as they began to move, the viewers could detect that the moving lights represented people, and even the emotional states of the various individuals came alive. In this way, it has been possible to demonstrate that the bright moving spots—called point-like displays—are sufficient for viewers to be able to determine, for example, the sex or emotional state of another person. Could it be that even inflammation, which could give you general clues about a person's state of health, influences a person's way of moving? In our first attempt at answering this question, people who received endotoxin or placebo simply walked down the hospital corridor while we filmed them. Other than walking speed, which we measured retrospectively from the films, we had no objective data, but used subjective impressions about how the people in the pictures were perceived by others. In fact, it turned out that this simple information from the film clips seemed to say something to the unknowing viewers: health is perceived as poorer, and people are judged to be more tired and slightly sadder, when they walk with a mild inflammation in their bodies. They also walk more slowly, something that was clearly related to how the subjects' health was perceived. As always in science, and not least with pioneering research, it is important to replicate results in order to exclude the possibility that randomness played a joke on us, or that our desire to find precisely these results influenced the process. In subsequent endotoxin experiments arranged by Julie Lasselin, blessed with organizational superpowers, we have now measured changes in gait patterns during inflammation using objective methods. People indeed walk more slowly, but also take shorter strides and have more rigid walking patterns. Interestingly, posture also changes, with a more downward-tilting head—quite similar to how sad or sick people have classically been depicted in art.

Overall, our behavior is important not only to regain health when we are ill, but also to avoid becoming ill at all. We are therefore sensitive to clues about the health of others, not only to avoid infection, but also to maximize our chances of passing on our genes. The mechanisms for detecting health cues in others are still largely unknown. The experiments we and others have done to date suggest that we share many strategies and communication systems with our animal peers in our quest to understand the health of others.

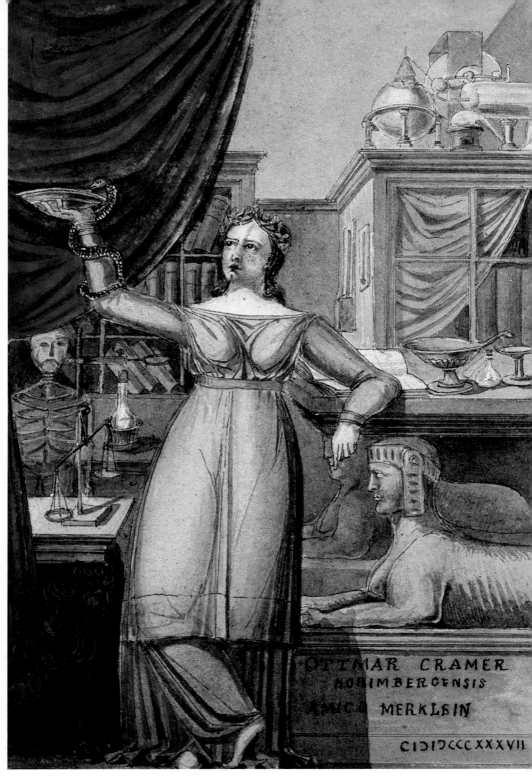

Hygieia, goddess of health, in a scientific cabinet

6

HOW DO YOU RATE YOUR GENERAL HEALTH?

What is the real meaning of the word "health"? Although health is so central to our everyday lives and livelihoods, it is difficult to define the concept. The Swedish National Encyclopedia offers the following bland description: "A difficult-to-define concept whose meaning extends beyond freedom from disease. A widely accepted definition is lacking."[1] An interesting but more extreme version is the World Health Organization's (WHO) classic definition from 1948: "Health is a state of complete physical, mental and social well-being and not merely the absence of disease or infirmity."[2] I doubt that even Jeanne Calment was completely healthy based on this definition.[3] The WHO's definition has been criticized for contributing to the medicalization of society, as total well-being in all these areas is difficult to achieve. In a way, WHO made us all into people with poor health. The definition can also be criticized because it does little to acknowledge the importance of functional ability in its focus on well-being. When it was published, the WHO's definition was still a novelty, as the concept included mental and social perspectives and not only the degree of disease. But what should one, then, include when defining the concept of health? If it is so tricky, can it be just as good to let individuals decide for themselves what they want to include in the

---

[1] https://www.ne.se/uppslagsverk/encyklopedi/lång/hälsa. Retrieved Sep 07 2021.
[2] https://www.who.int/about/governance/constitution. Retrieved Sep 07 2021.
[3] Calment lived until she was 122, despite smoking during a period of her life (but only between the ages of 21 and 117). Calment's longevity has however been questioned based on the suspicion that her daughter Yvonne may have assumed her identity in 1934.

The Inflamed Feeling. Mats Lekander, Oxford University Press. © Mats Lekander 2022.
DOI: 10.1093/oso/9780198863441.003.0006

definition? In any case, this is what has been done in a large number of scientific studies: using a single and extremely simplified question about health without specifying what is really meant. As we shall see, it has been a successful strategy.

Health as seen through a crystal ball

One of the most common questions in health-related research is this: In general, how would you rate your health? The response is usually stated as a scale of response options, from very poor to very good, and is common in sociological, epidemiological, medical, and psychological research. While the question is one of the most widely used, it is also one of the least understood. What do we really mean, and why does the rating provide all the information it has been shown to do?

Self-estimates of health were included in large studies during the 1970s and 1980s when it was not feasible to conduct regular health surveys of all study participants. Could one instead just ask the person how he or she viewed their health? To the surprise of many, it was later found that self-rated health was among the best, if not the best, research questions to accurately predict death. It was at the same level or better than diagnosis or medication, thus objectively measurable factors. When statistically adjusted for somatic or psychiatric illnesses, age, socioeconomic status, gender, medication, and similar factors, the predictive power decreased somewhat, but was still convincingly strong and statistically significant by a broad margin.

Wondrous findings, which have since been repeated many times. A few years ago, a new study was published that also attracted great attention among researchers. The authors of the study investigated how mortality within a five-year period could be predicted by using information in the UK Biobank, which includes about 500,000 people. There are several differences between this and previous studies. The study is very large and can therefore provide a reliable estimate of how strong the relationships really are. You can also divide the material into different groups and see, for example, how mortality in cardiovascular disease is best predicted in comparison to overall mortality. Another advantage is the number of factors included in the material: more than five hundred so-called predictors (that is, something that could predict the likelihood of something happening in the future), meaning that information from questionnaires and those obtained from biological tests can be compared. What was the best predictor for mortality? For men it was self-rated health. For women, self-rated health was the fourth best predictor, close to two questions about cancer and one about recent illness or injury. This is in competition with over five hundred other predictors. Another strong predictor of mortality, even stronger than smoking and other lifestyle measures, was self-reported walking speed. Self-rated health and walking speed were, in our studies, both negatively affected by inflammatory activation, as I described earlier.

An interesting finding relates to which general type of measurement could best predict mortality. It turned out to be the type of information you get by asking people questions. Responses to these questions in this large study were thus better than biomedical measurements, such as measures based on blood sampling[4] or other tests. Thus, the human brain contains a wealth of information that can be combined and summarized in the answer to a single question, a response that may say more than the results of many refined biological measurement methods. Some of the information available to the brain relates to knowledge about diagnoses, hereditary diseases, parents' lifespan, or other factors of a biomedical nature. Another part concerns the feeling of health. Do you feel healthy? How do you view your health right now? How do you usually perceive your health to be?

Findings from the UK Biobank confirm those from many other previous studies showing the relationship between self-rated health and mortality in many countries; in different age groups; in patients with cardiovascular disease, cancer, or other chronic conditions; in individuals with acute

---

[4] Note that factors such as lipids were not measured.

health conditions; or in the general population. The way in which the question is asked or how the answer is given varies to some extent, but the connection is still stable over these different versions.

Not surprisingly, self-rated health also predicts objective health measures other than mortality. These include morbidity, healthcare consumption, and sick leave. I should clarify here that these relationships, as usual, have been shown to be consistent at the group level. And I am well aware that you as a reader (and I as a writer) do not necessarily feel that you are in mint condition at any given moment or even for long periods. But in any case, if we study a number of people with poorer self-rated health and adjust the relationship for other factors (such as diagnosis), they have an increased risk of future objective ill health. But there will be plenty of exceptions. Individuals with good self-rated health who become ill or die prematurely, and individuals with poor self-rated health who remain fit as a fiddle (from the perspective of not having any verifiable disease). This discrepancy is itself quite interesting. Some people with diagnoses for serious illnesses, who have a long list of medications or poor test outcomes, still think their health is good. Why? In these cases too there is a reduced risk of further future ill health compared to people with the same objective health status, but poorer subjective health. And others are constantly worrying about being sick, even though they are actually healthy.

Since self-rated health has been shown to be so important from the perspectives of both suffering and objective health, and is a cheap and **easy measurement to use, the question is sometimes included in clinical** trials that evaluate treatments. In general clinical care, a systematic use of self-ratings of health has not been implemented, but a change may be underway. As we shall see later, there are many forces that are now working to better utilize patients' perspectives in a systematic way. Once again, hard facts support the use of subjective input: important information can be obtained from subjective data that can be linked to quantifiable outcomes, and perhaps to the most quantifiable of all—money.

Why you perceive your health as good or poor

Self-rated health is an inclusive measure in that the person responding to the question is affected by, and takes a position on, a large number of factors before even choosing to answer "very good." What influences this choice? The measure is not only inclusive but also individual, so that different types of information are given different weight depending on who you are. Maybe function—being able to do the things you think are important in life even though your legs may hurt and your eyelids feel heavy—is especially important for one person, while the absence of diagnosed illness is given greater weight by another person. Since self-rated health is subjective and evaluative in this way, it is difficult to define exactly what it really is. How could it be anything but subjective, and how could the same things be appraised in the same way across individuals? Each person creates his or her own interpretive framework because it is not specified what is really meant by health. This means that each individual answers the question based on the meaning they derive from areas that are important to them, and also from positive factors that might easily be missed. Could the fact that individuals consider aspects that they personally deem important contribute to the predictive power of personal health assessments? It cannot be excluded, but it is not easy to prove. If people did not include important things, the predictive power would not be as strong, that's for sure. It is also reasonable to assume that there is not only a quantitative difference between the response options (from very poor to very good), but that there is also a qualitative difference between good and poor health. The Finnish philosopher Georg Henrik von Wright argued that good health is a normal condition that need not be explained, and that it is its exception, poor health, that we need to explain and justify. The phrase "no news is good news," or that good health keeps quiet, describes this approach, and suggests the surprise we feel when some part of the body suddenly does not function properly. Why did I take its functionality for granted, and why did I not appreciate it before it began to cause me problems?

Nevertheless, it is possible to conclude that certain factors are of particular importance to most people when making a subjective health assessment. These include symptoms that, for most of you reading this book, or for most people with a body, are not surprising: fatigue, depressed mood, and pain. Functional factors, such as memory and fitness, are important. Psychosocial factors related to home, family, or leisure may also have significance. The findings I have summarized here are based on Swedish surveys and other studies where large groups of people were asked to rate their health and at the same time answer a number of other questions. When similar surveys have been carried out in extensive studies of British civil servants and employees of the French gas and electric company, overlapping results have been obtained. The most important ones were symptom load, sick leave, and some measures of mental and physical health. An interesting finding from the French survey was that physical fatigue was by far most strongly associated with participants' self-rated health. This is in line with other studies that show that short or poor sleep is associated with poor self-rated health. But the studies also show differences between groups of people. It is likely that the more physically strenuous work that the French electricity and gas workers experienced, in comparison with the British civil servants, meant that physical fatigue varied more and for statistical reasons therefore had more power to explain variation in self-rated health. Circumstances, of course, play an important role when examining the relative influence that key factors have on phenomena we are trying to understand. If the UK study group was less fatigued (and varied less in the level of fatigue between individuals), the statistical relationship with self-rated health would have been weaker.[5]

---

[5] I draw particular attention to this because it illustrates a pedagogical problem that is often present in the interaction between research and society. As an example, in folk psychology and among management consultants, it is often claimed that 93 percent of the information in a conversation consists of non-verbal information. The statement is too general to say anything at all, and the amount of non-verbal information must in fact vary

A separate study of Finnish and Italian people within the general population examined similar questions. The study found that having fewer symptoms, fewer illnesses, better functioning, and better education were associated with better self-rated health. These findings were found to be valid in both Finland (Tampere) and Italy (Florence), but in this study the effect was also linked to gender and nationality. In fact, it was several times more likely that a woman or man in Florence described themselves as being in good health compared to a man living in Tampere. It is reasonable that cultural differences in how one responds (for example, the likelihood that one does not wish to tempt fate by claiming that one's health is very good) affect results, not only "true" differences in perceived health.

All in all, it is clear that health is perceived as a much more complex concept than just the absence of illness, which in that sense is consistent with the WHO definition described earlier. Recent studies have even shown the role that emotions play, and how particularly positive emotional expressions contribute to better self-rated health. This is interesting because positive emotions are not just the absence of negative ones, so they should therefore have beneficial subjective health effects even in tough times that are dominated by negative emotions. Whether this means that it is good from a health perspective to initiate activities that make you experience positive emotions is not entirely clear, but it is a reasonable

widely in different situations, for example, depending on whether or not you can see each other when speaking. But if that were generally true, it would be great for those who dislike studying foreign languages—the ability to converse when traveling abroad could only increase by a maximum of 7 percent! Ninety-three percent of the information would still be conveyed. Another example that illustrates the importance of context is borrowed from the answer to a viewer's question during a television program: How much of a chameleon's color is determined by genetic factors and how much by its environment? The expert answer was: it depends. The viewer was instructed to imagine that the animal's color is studied in an environment of homogeneous color, thus with minimal influence on the animal's color. The amount of variation that can be explained by genetic factors will then be much larger than in an environment of varying colors, since the environment in which the animal was studied would not stimulate color changes. Against a backdrop of varying colors, the environment would exert greater influence. One should add, however, that it is actually the octopus, not the chameleon, that is particularly skilled at changing color based on the background.

interpretation. If nothing else, you can experience the enjoyment and get an emotional boost during difficult times, even if it is only temporary.

This tells us that to *feel* healthy, it is good if you are free from illness in the biomedical sense, but that a number of other factors also contribute substantially. This applies to knowledge about illnesses, sick leave, accidents, functional ability or disability, or the absence of such factors, which can all affect how you appraise your health. But it is also about how you feel at the moment, and how you usually feel. Whether one has a tangible feeling of health or not in the body, experiences more positive or negative emotions, or is satisfied with one's life situation—such factors all affect one's subjective, or self-rated, health status.

A study of 407 randomly selected Stockholm adults compared the individuals' self-rated health with physicians' assessments of their health. The physicians' assessments were based on the individuals' physical health including specific health problems, medication, and blood tests. Social problems were not included. The information was summarized along a five-point scale ranging from good to poor health. The medical estimates were consistent with the patients' estimates in approximately 60 percent of cases. The moderate agreement again says something about the importance of factors that lie outside the classic biomedical health model in people's own health ratings. In fact, psychosocial factors, such as mental and social well-being, were those that were most strongly related to how participants rated their health. In a relatively large number of cases, the doctors' and patients' estimates actually contradicted one another. It is worth noting here that we do not know the extent to which the physicians' estimates would have been influenced by the patients' overall situation if they had not been instructed to focus strictly on their physical health; the instruction likely made the doctors ignore psychosocial cues to a greater extent than normal.

The scale used for self-rated health usually spans from very poor to very good health, often in five steps. So is "very poor" the worst thing imaginable in terms of perceived health? There is a neurological/psychiatric disorder that I would claim is even worse than "very poor health," namely

Cotard's syndrome (or "walking corpse syndrome"),[6] in which sufferers believe they are dead. It has aptly been called "a disease of human health."

Are subjective health ratings used in healthcare?

The answer to this question is not the resounding "yes" that one might think. If subjective complaints prompt people to frequently seek healthcare, one can assume that it is easy to measure the extent to which the problems decrease following (often expensive) treatment. In many cases, the subjective factors overlap with healthcare goals such as reducing symptoms like chronic pain, or minimizing the negative impact of chronic pain on patients' lives despite medical treatment. So once again, why not measure? In fact, a change is underway in the form of an international movement to systematically collect so-called patient-reported outcome measures (see Chapter 8). Such measures have often been included in clinical research, but in healthcare they have primarily taken the form of patient satisfaction, which only provides a limited perspective. Other questions try to capture the "values" that healthcare has delivered to patients. These benefits are easier to measure if you systematically collect data on symptoms, functional ability, health behaviors, and quality of life. Taking such values into account can play an important role in achieving health outcomes and reducing healthcare time, but more and better research on benefits is sorely needed.

This increased interest in patient-reported outcomes will move healthcare closer to the perspective I have presented in this book—subjective factors should be included and combined with biological factors, and they should be measured objectively (with validated methods) and seen as the

---

[6] Cotard's syndrome was named after the French nineteenth-century neurologist Jules Cotard who first described the condition. It is characterized by bodily delusions such as the loss of body parts or denial of their own existence. Curiously, a number of Cotard's syndrome cases have been reported as side effects of treatment with Aciclovir, a drug used to treat the herpes virus.

important indicators that they are. According to some calculations, both suffering and social costs can be reduced.

Why is perceived health such a strong indicator of future health?

If self-rated health is such a good predictor of future objective health, then why is it so? The short answer is that we don't know. Personally, I became interested in understanding the mechanisms behind self-rated health after seeing this 1998 statement from the Swedish Research Council Board: "Several studies have shown that the subjective perception of poor health can be an important early warning sign about future medically detectable morbidity and mortality." [7]Extraordinarily interesting, I thought. How might that work? And why was subjective perception so powerful?

Naturally, the more that is known about objective health factors for a group you study over time, the less self-rated health will contribute in terms of independent explanatory power. Will this share of self-rated health's explanatory power gradually diminish as better objective outcome measures become available and are implemented in routine care or research? It is unlikely that the share of explained variation in mortality, for example, will shrink to an insignificant crumb. The reason I believe this is that the brain's ability to pull together relevant information of both an external (knowledge about one's life) and internal (feelings related to the body) nature is hard to beat. In addition, our subjective health estimates affect how we behave and in turn our objective health. According to a large American study, the relationship between self-rated health and mortality has actually become stronger compared to 30 years ago. Increased information and knowledge about health may be a possible cause of this increase in explanatory power.

---

[7] Forskningsrådsnämnden, Rapport 98:7.

Thus, there appear to be two main explanations that can contribute to subjective health estimates' prediction of future health. The first explanation can be called "accurate." The estimate we make is to some extent a correct assessment of our current health situation. The second explanation can be called "causal," due to the fact that our behavior can be positively affected when we consider ourselves to be healthier, or vice versa.

Many of the factors that affect how we perceive our health are not stable over time. This applies, of course, to illnesses that may come and go, but in addition, health behaviors can change (we may sleep less for some time and feel less healthy), as well as our social or economic circumstances. Furthermore, neither symptoms like pain, fatigue, or depression nor positive emotions are stable over time. They can vary within hours, days, or weeks when we work extra hard and steal sleep time or stress out over an exam. They can also vary along with long-term life changes when we move, divorce, change health behaviors, marry, develop new interests, fall in love, change jobs, start to exercise, worry excessively, or read too many exaggerated articles about health problems.

Because self-rated health is sensitive to so many changing aspects of health or living conditions, it should also change as circumstances change. This is also the case. Can changes in subjective health perception also affect how well it predicts future objective illness? The answer is yes; in cases in which there has been a change in participant's ratings, the predictive power has improved as compared to when only a single measurement has been used in the prediction.

Thus, there appears to be a stable part of self-rated health that changes slowly or very little, and another part that is sensitive to shorter changes and daily condition. A simple analogy is to compare the stable part with "climate" and the changing part with "weather." How do you rate the climate where you live? To what extent do you think you are assessing the climate differently depending on whether you make the judgment on a rainy day or a sunny day? It is likely that you rate the climate as better if you assess it on a sunny day (unless you are a professional or recreational farmer and have just experienced a period of drought, belong to the group of rain fans, or are plagued by the tiring effects of pollen allergy on the brain). This is probably similar with health estimates—a more variable part and a more stable one, but where daily conditions shape how we perceive the stable, long-term part. "Current health" affects how we assess our overall state of health.

If you read too many leaflets with frightening health messages; too many alarming claims about the connections between sleep, stress, and health; or reports about the high proportion of mental illness in the population and its contribution to sick leave, you can imagine that we are on the slippery slope. The truth is in fact that our health, both objectively and subjectively, is becoming gradually better rather than worse. In Sweden and many other countries, life expectancy has increased over the last decades. In the UK as well as the USA, the increase has however slowed (and small declines have even been noted in recent years).

Those with a college education who have reached the age of 30 have now even longer to think about whether they (really) are healthy, before health becomes both an objective and subjective concern. This example points to the important inequalities in health, a view reinforced by the fact that the worst development in average life expectancy has been seen in women with only a primary or lower secondary education.

But we feel worse now, under such troublesome conditions, right? No, in fact not. In terms of self-rated health, the change is the same as for our general increase in average life expectancy, and has thus improved. In fact, far less than 10 percent of the populations in the UK, Sweden, or the USA rate their health as bad or very bad. However, good health is not equally distributed. Men are generally more likely to respond that their health is good than women. Also, more people with higher levels of education indicate that their health is good, and younger people rate their health as good more often than the elderly.

Most studies investigating self-rated health—and there have been quite a few—have been done by observing people in the general population, measuring cross-sectional relationships at one moment in time, or over a period of time (such as when predicting the risk of death over a five-year period based on a subjective health estimate). Remember the mantra "association is not causation." But few studies have been done with an experimental control where one manipulates a factor that is believed to affect self-rated health. In these cases, self-rated health can be compared with that of an untreated control group, or with a different time period for the same person that has not been manipulated. If we believe that we understand the factors that have the greatest influence on most people's self-rated health, we would want to be able to manipulate them and confirm whether or not the subjective health experience is affected by the change. We have recently been able to conduct such studies in which we influenced two favorite factors (sleep and inflammation) to see if health appraisal changed as a result of manipulation.

In a study led by John Axelsson, we measured some healthy (I would even say very healthy, since they volunteer to participate in studies involving hardships) people's sleep over a longer period of time. We were interested in sleep because sleep duration and sleep quality, energy level, and fatigue have been shown to be related to self-rated health. After following the participants for some time, they were instructed to switch from sleeping eight hours a night to just four hours a night for five days. The effect of the manipulation thus corresponded to a hard week of work with far too little time for recovery. Four hours a night is very little sleep for most, but not unreasonably short. Each day, the study participants filled out several questionnaires that included a question on self-rated health. Since we were interested in daily changes, we asked participants to evaluate their health "that day" rather than their general state of health. The result was clear. After the first day with too little sleep, participants' self-rated health deteriorated noticeably, and then a little more for each extra day of sleep deprivation (see Figure 6.1). After only a few nights of recovery sleep (normal sleep), health assessments returned to the level they started with. Self-ratings of health declined as the subjects felt more tired, and it was likely that the persistent fatigue (see Figure 6.1) mainly made the participants appraise their health as increasingly worse as sleep deprivation increased. It may sound like an obvious conclusion, but let's

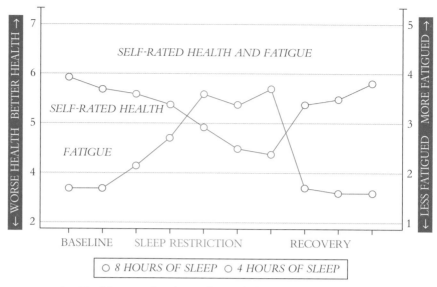

FIGURE 6.1 Health is rated as lower for each day with insufficient sleep, concurrently with increases in fatigue.

remember that many factors can affect self-rated health, and sleep deprivation can have several consequences that can also affect subjective perceived health. One of these is increased pain, or increased pain sensitivity, to which sleep loss can contribute.

It may be worth pointing out that in the short term, being careless about sleep is hardly unhealthy, but it surely does not make you feel healthier. Sleep deprivation has emotional consequences that, in addition to fatigue, is likely to contribute to making one's health feel worse. One of the consequences of too little sleep and fatigue is that you look less favorably on life, nudging you toward a dystopic view, which probably includes health. When you have slept too little, you may assume that the heavy feeling you have in your body and your negative mood are typical for you and not just a valid reaction to the situation. This is a type of bias or distorted thinking—in this case, that a temporary negative mood affects one's general health assessment. There are, as I said, very few studies that actively try to influence how health is appraised, but in some instances we have also tried to directly influence a biological system involved in sending reports on health processes from the body to the brain. The immune system is central to such processes, so what happens to the feeling of health if you stimulate the immune system?

The body's sickness signals

In Chapter 4 on the sickness response, I described a communication system that affects the brain and how we feel when we get sick. As you recall, it was about inflammation products—cytokines—that influence the brain's activity so that we develop a fever, feel tired, and depressed, and experience a sore and pain-sensitive body. The desire for and pleasure from many different "external" activities decreases, and all this is believed to be a way for the overall immune defense to increase the chance of survival. We reduce the level of risk that external active behaviors can entail and reduce the use of energy that is instead used for fever and for the activity of the white blood cells.

The symptoms of an inflammatory reaction are clearly similar to the symptoms that are strongly associated with poor self-rated health. In spite of this, our research group noted early on that no systematic attempts to link the degree of inflammatory activity to the level of self-rated health had been made. Before I describe how we performed such studies, and finally started manipulating the immune system by giving endotoxin (the method I described in Chapter 4) to see how healthy people's health assessments are affected, I want to remind you of an aspect of inflammatory activity that is easily overlooked. When the immune system detects a foreign substance that seeks to invade our bodies, a number of defense mechanisms become activated. This can result not only in local inflammation (a place on the body that swells, turns red, and aches) but also systemic inflammation, and inflammatory products spread in the blood, which also affect the brain and behavior. This is elementary classic immunology, at least if you exclude the effects on the brain. But as the field of immunology has been forced into general physiology and is decreasingly seen as an isolated academic subject or biological system, it has been recognized that the inflammatory substances have important regulatory functions even under healthy conditions. The cytokines, for example, are included in such diverse functions as the regulation of sleep, formation of long-term memory, and metabolism. This is not surprising in itself—available substances tend to appear in different places and systems, and do "double duty" when the genetic code to produce these substances is available. In other words, this part of the inflammatory system is not simply "off" or "on" but is constantly active to some degree in different parts of the body. For example, cytokines participate when long-term memories—such as when you learn new words and remember their meaning—are created, and these molecules must therefore be available even in a person without infection or obvious illness. All in all, this means that one can measure low levels of inflammatory "markers" in anyone's blood. Above this basic physiological level, mild increases in inflammatory signals in the blood have been shown to be involved in disease processes that previously were not thought to involve inflammation at all, such as subtypes of depression, schizophrenia, or some pain conditions. To describe such processes, the term "low-grade inflammation" has grown common. But a mild increase in inflammatory products is also linked to how you feel, what you want to do, and what you actually do.

With these observations in mind, it didn't seem far-fetched that variations in inflammatory activity could be related to how you appraise your health. First of all, we wanted to understand mechanisms that explain appraisal of (general) health. To investigate the relationships of interest, we needed both to collect blood samples and to ask health-related questions, and also consider a substantial number of control variables for a large number of people. In the first study, we examined individuals who came to a primary care unit in Hallonbergen, outside of Stockholm. The individuals' health varied in expected ways, from generally healthy (but who still occasionally seek out primary care) to quite ill. Together with researcher Anna Andreasson, we have, in several subsequent studies, investigated patients with cardiovascular disease, a representative sample of people from the general population in Sweden, approximately 47,000 young men examined during military conscription, and a sample of elderly generally healthy Americans. In these studies, we observed an association between higher levels of (some measure of) inflammation and poorer self-rated health. The relationship remained when we statistically adjusted for (or excluded) those with an objectively diagnosed disease or who regularly take medication. It therefore appears that a mild inflammatory response is associated with a poorer health experience. As is usually the case in research, the results vary slightly from study to study, and in the first study of primary care patients, for example, we only saw the relationship in women and could not confirm it in the relatively few participating men. One particularly interesting result was that the relationship between inflammation and self-rated health was much stronger than between inflammation and the "biomedical" health rating performed by the primary care physician. As a researcher with a particular interest in subjective health experiences, this was a very exciting result that I hope to replicate and follow up on. When we placed the subjective health experiences in a theoretically coherent perspective, the results generated interest and prompted many other research groups to investigate the same relationship with similar methods in other populations, which is what we encourage in research, so that we can trust the findings. The pattern of results has been confirmed (as always with some variation) in, for example, studies of older Americans (other than the ones we examined), in Japanese students, and in other groups.

In future studies, researchers need to follow people over time, including those who receive treatment for mental or somatic ill health, to see if inflammation is involved in the causal chain between self-rated health and future mortality. In our study with older Americans, we measured the relationship between an inflammatory variable (interleukin-6, the cytokine most commonly studied in relation to self-rated health) and self-rated health a total of 10 times. On every occasion we saw a connection between higher inflammation and relatively poorer self-rated health. However, as a humble servant of truth and education, I want to point out that, as usual, the relationship explains only a limited part of the connection. This means that the inflammation explains a certain part of the variation in self-rated health, but far from all.

Taken together, most studies show that higher levels of inflammatory cytokines are generally linked to poorer self-rated health. The relationships also remain when statistically adjusted for detectable disease or other factors. Adjusting a relationship means that the statistical calculation takes into account a factor that could otherwise explain the relationship. For example, it could be that people with diabetes have both poorer health and higher levels of inflammation, without the inflammation having a true effect on the health experience.

The results thus far support our theoretical assumptions that inflammatory products carry health-relevant information to the brain and affect its activity level.

But a methodological caveat must be noted. If we only measure how things relate to one another, and mostly in cross-sectional analyses with measurements made at one point in time, then we cannot conclude anything about causality. What affects what? Maybe there is some genetic factor that makes people who feel unhealthy also have higher inflammatory activity? Or is it the perception of poor health that contributes to higher inflammatory activity because it is interpreted as a threat? The latter is conceivable because, for example, stress-related hormones involved in the stress response can activate genes in white blood cells and cause them to increase the production of inflammatory substances. Perhaps it is doubtful that the effect would be so strong that it would appear in all these studies in the way that it has, but to know whether higher inflammation can directly affect self-rated health, experimentally controlled studies are needed in which individuals are randomized to receive either something that stimulates the immune system or a placebo. And that's exactly what we did in the studies where we gave endotoxin to humans, as I described in Chapter 4 on the sickness response.

Focusing on the sick body

I described earlier how the rating of health can be framed within a shorter time period so that it corresponds to "current" health. Not surprisingly, this health estimate drops dramatically about an hour after receiving endotoxin compared to pre-injection or placebo. We have also investigated this with different doses of endotoxin, and have seen quite clearly that with higher doses the effect increases. What is baffling, however, is what happens to general health assessments. It turns out that participants rated their general health as significantly worse after the endotoxin stimulated an inflammatory response, despite the fact that they stated prior to receiving endotoxin that they considered their general health to be very good. Could asking about their general health several times have prompted them to alter their later responses to an answer they believed we expected? To avoid this possibility, at one point (when the volunteers had received a slightly lower dose) we asked them only once, after the endotoxin had been in their systems for an hour and a half, and compared the results with the people who received a placebo (see Figure 6.2). The result was equally clear, albeit slightly weaker, probably because the dose was slightly lower. We could therefore conclude that inflammation affected the perceived health levels of the individuals. Overall, the effect was very strong. The individuals were perfectly healthy but changed their health assessments so that, on average, they corresponded to that of the primary care patients we previously discussed. Although the individuals we injected with endotoxin were young and had no chronic illnesses (older people generally tend to judge their health to be slightly worse than younger people do), they now stated that their general state of health was at the same level as a group of older patients, a majority of whom had specific health complaints.

Is there a "switch" that can be adjusted so that when we get sick, one's attention is more focused on the body than on the outside world? Can it be activated by stress, insufficient sleep, or lack of social context? Can it, like other functions, be trained through excessive attention to the body?

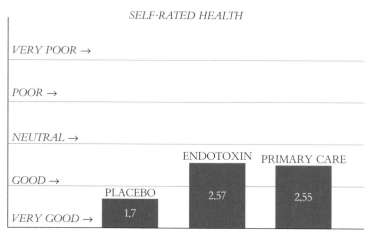

FIGURE 6.2 Self-rated general health 90 minutes after healthy young people (average age less than 30 years) were injected with placebo (bar 1) or endotoxin (bar 2), compared to primary care patients (average age less than 60 years) at a healthcare center in Stockholm, Sweden (bar 3). Of the primary care patients, some had no diagnosis at all, while others had chronic diseases. The figure shows that healthy young people estimated their health as worse after they received endotoxin, at the same level as middle-aged patients in primary care.

Inspired from Bianka Karshikoff

Can increased time and opportunity to consider "how the body feels" help overactivate a function in the brain (increased inward attention) and thereby aggravate or even create problems in itself? Do we boost such a function by constantly asking others and our children how they feel or how they slept? Perhaps the latter kind of questions help us more easily note deviations from the expected norm, a condition we learned to associate with the absence of illness and ailments, and with total physical, mental, and social well-being. Under these circumstances, it is easy to feel ill, and to perceive things happening in the body as symptoms of ill health.

A switch like the one I described has yet to be found, although many illnesses seem to be associated with the fact that we pay more attention to and worry about our body's condition. We notice aches and fatigue, we notice discomfort and malaise, and we may have butterflies in our stomachs. These phenomena also apply to acute illnesses, such as when we have a proper cold. If we succeed in drawing attention to something outside of ourselves (we may have gone to work even though it felt like a hardship), we may forget about the cold and suddenly realize, "Oh right, I'm sick. But how nice not to think about it for a while."

There may be one or more functions in the brain that switch our balance of attention from "outward" to "inward" when we are ill. Some observations support this notion. As the researcher Predrag Petrovic has concluded, there are some signs that the regulation of interoceptive (which deals with the inner world) and exteroceptive (from the outside world) information compete with each other. In fact, areas for receiving and controlling internal and external information are found side by side in the brain. They also seem to inhibit each other. The current areas are part of different networks that, during rest, inhibit one another's activity; this can be seen among subjects who are resting in an MRI scanner without performing any specific tasks. To some extent, the size and degree of activity in these brain areas can differ between people with different types of mental illness. In these types of illnesses, people find it difficult to regulate information either from the inner or the outer world. In practical terms, this means that some people can be sensitive to and easily disturbed by signals from the inner world or from the outer world.

Inflammatory activation is hypothesized, but not yet proven, to contribute to increased awareness of the inner world, and to increase the discomfort and affective response from symptoms such as pain. It has however been shown that attention to external factors, and controlling this attention, is impaired by inflammatory activity. A large number of studies have shown that inflammation in response to bacterial substances increases the insula's activity, which supports the idea that inflammation contributes to focusing more attention on the body. This probably contributes to increased attention to the body when you are ill, and to the general feeling of deteriorating health.

If we have a body that constantly shouts "hello!"—a bit like the barking dog or meowing cat that is hard to ignore—it is no wonder if we focus attention inward rather than outward. But if it is true that the interoception "volume" becomes louder during illness, it would be fantastic if we could adjust it for people whose attention is "stuck" in the inward position. In fact, cognitive behavioral therapy often includes techniques that support focus on outward rather than inward attention. Behaviors that are rewarding over the long term are encouraged, even if the body protests, and to learn to accept bodily symptoms so that they do not require attention and hinder other activities. This can include measures to reduce the fear of pain and thereby the fear of movement that triggers the pain. In interoceptive terms, this would correspond to assigning a lower fear value to the pain signal. With a lower fear value, the corresponding behavioral response (to keep still) weakens, which otherwise becomes a problem for people trying to lead a satisfying life. It is possible that the feeling of discomfort may decrease at the same time, even if the pain signal is perceived as equally strong.

In everyday speech you may hear the term "enhanced perception," when you pay particular attention to something in which you have a special interest. I think most people recognize the phenomenon from when they have recently become interested in something, perhaps a certain style of hat, a dog breed, or a car model—we suddenly see these objects wherever we turn. The thing we have become interested in seems to have become more common and shows up everywhere. Our new interest can, of course, affect the attention we pay to the object in question so that we notice it at every opportunity, and it is also coded into our memory. The object penetrates the noise.

In psychology, the phenomenon of "selective attention" has long been of interest and is often exemplified by the so-called "cocktail party effect." If we are in a group of people at a cocktail party or in a similar context, we can usually easily follow what a conversation partner is saying, despite the fact that many others are talking at the same time. You don't hear what the others are saying. But if your own name is mentioned, you suddenly notice the other conversation, even though you were apparently unaware of it before you heard your name. Your attention shifts from the conversation you were engaged in to the one in which your name was mentioned, since the signal value for one's own name is so strong. Thus to some extent, we heard the other conversations, even though they were filtered out and did not reach our consciousness, or remained for a few seconds as a brief memory like decaying, unattended echoes.

It is reasonable to assume that one could temporarily, or for an extended time, increase the value of bodily signals. This means that there is an additional similarity between ordinary perception of the surrounding world (that is, exteroception) and perception of our inner world (or interoception). According to the filter theory, all information from the outside world must pass through two filtering systems if we are to become aware of it. The first is a sensory system and the second, a central perceptual system. In the sensory system, information can only be retained for a limited time. The perceptual system selects the information we attended to. Thus, there is an automatic screening or filtering function that allows only certain information to be collected, stored, and processed. Other information is neglected and constitutes noise.

For a person with a chronic illness, aches, fatigue, stiffness, and other health-related signals appear to be among the information that can be selected and chosen for selective attention. Sometimes the term "somatic amplification" is used, which is considered to be associated with certain disease states, such as depression. The term stands for the tendency of bodily stimuli, like pain or tiredness, to be "amplified" and exert greater influence than normal.

For a person with plenty of opportunity to ponder their inner state, it may be hard for internal signals to become overridden and replaced by impressions from the outside world. A therapist can take advantage of this phenomenon. A person in acute crisis, with unbearable feelings and thoughts and who is at risk of self-harm, may be asked to carefully look at the surroundings and reproduce them. "What does it look like where you are?" "Describe details and everything you see in the immediate area," a care provider may urge. If the method succeeds, the new information can "take over" and reduce the unbearable feelings and the imminent threat. Does the technique remind you about how to comfort a child who has hurt themselves? After a while, it's time to point the child's attention toward something other than the pain. You may need to get the child to see something in the environment or be interested in something fun that will happen. If it works, the pain is suddenly filtered away and disappears from the available conscious workspace. The flashlight that constitutes consciousness is steered in a different direction, and the pain disappears from the narrow beam of light and into the darkness—gone, or at least severely weakened.

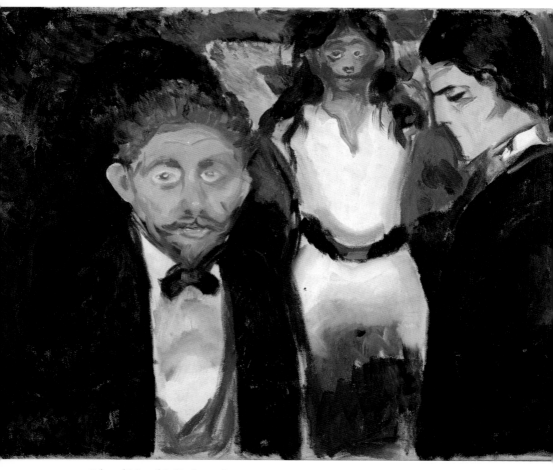

Edvard Munch's "Jealousy"
Luisa Ricciarini/Bridgeman Images

7

FEELING SICK AND OTHER EMOTIONS

Is health like an emotion? A feeling of being sick or not, seen in the broad perspective, in which both the feeling of the body and factors such as social security and functional ability are weighed in? The experiential and affective aspect is obvious, in addition to the more cognitive assessment that is made when considering the presence of a diagnosis or other factors. In psychology and neuroscience, knowledge about emotions is a cornerstone for understanding human behavior and mental health. An emotion is a reaction pattern that is activated in response to events that are relevant to us, for example to our goals, to what is important and urgent, or to our safety. The emotions then guide further cognitive processes such as perception, attention, memory, and judgments. If these responses take place in systems that have the capacity for consciousness, conscious experiences—or what we commonly call "feelings"—arise. In the same way that other emotions can become an all too typical response pattern—individuals with anxiety disorders, for example, have internal systems for fear and anxiety that are too easily and too often activated—it turns out that low-grade inflammation and easily triggered disease responses are part of the problem in both somatic and mental health. The sickness response is, in fact, very similar to a classic emotion, and the frequency with which we feel that we are sick may be part of what we view as our general state of health.

The Inflamed Feeling. Mats Lekander, Oxford University Press. © Mats Lekander 2022.
DOI: 10.1093/oso/9780198863441.003.0007

How the brain processes signals from the outer and inner worlds

A central element of this book is that psychological and evolutionary perspectives can be applied to better understand areas that traditionally belong to biology and medicine. While a lot has happened over the past decade, using this approach to understand and better manage several common healthcare problems is still an open target. Perception psychology, with its long-standing and successful tradition of analyzing function and "laws" of organization, has been tremendously helpful in understanding the brain. The same psychology of perception is slowly helping us chart ways of understanding our bodies and the signals it sends. The underlying logic is that the systems that understand external events are similar to those that understand internal events. Both systems must select important information at the expense of other. Both systems must be able to actively pay attention to certain information, pay special attention to changes, and figure things out well in advance to be able to prepare and sometimes start activity even before something happens. They must "guess" and use past experience to put as little computational power as possible into the task. The need to dynamically control the functions is also common to both systems. And finally, all these normal functions can be dysregulated so that problems arise and the "borders" of an illness may be crossed.

Borders of an illness—what would that be? Well we all, for example, have an anxiety system with fluctuating levels to deal with, where social evaluation—what others think of us and our achievements—is one of the threats to be addressed. For most people, this kind of threat is clearly felt and is experienced as nervousness before and during sensitive occasions. But when the occasion, perhaps the presentation of a project at school or work, is over, the anxiety is also over. The task was carried out in the presence of the negative emotion, followed by a sense of relief, and the next time, or perhaps the time after that, the anxiety diminished and you became accustomed to the situation. No disaster occurred, and it probably won't in the future either. This is called habituation. The system is necessary for us to consider situations and threats that may occur, so that we can prepare and allocate a reasonable level of resources to urgent tasks. But for some people, the danger of social evaluation—the scrutiny from schoolmates or colleagues—feels so severe that anxiety becomes unreasonably strong. What signs of negative evaluation can be detected in the audience? Critical facial expressions? Someone who looks tired or is about to fall asleep, arms crossed, and body language expressing skepticism? Laughter as the audience entered the room that was probably aimed at you? The anxiety is so strong that avoidance becomes the natural response, as far as possible. When the threat has subsided, rumination over what happened or concern for the next evaluation takes over. When this makes life difficult to handle, it is called social phobia—a normal function that is dysregulated and reaches such disabling levels that it meets diagnostic criteria and is given a name; that is, the person "has" the diagnosis. Perceptual and emotional systems needed to motivate and change behavior can be dysregulated, cause great difficulties, and then be described with—now crossing the border—the epithet "illness."

These types of control functions with the potential to become dysregulated are common to external and internal stimuli. I am not saying in any way that it is the person's own fault. I say that normal systems that make us more or less sensitive to something, such as pain (the need for pain inhibition varies from one situation to another), can be regulated in a dysfunctional way. Other examples of systems that can be dysregulated are attention to external factors (such as in attention deficit hyperactivity disorder (ADHD), where external factors attract attention too easily), instability and excessive attention to internal factors and emotions (like in cases of borderline personality disorder), or attention to bodily changes and the risk of becoming ill (hypochondriasis or health anxiety). The boundary between sick and healthy becomes a matter of definition, and it is not necessarily so that people are sick or healthy in an obvious way. All of the described functions are examples of emotional systems that are prepared to help us appropriately control behavior. How they vary between and within people suggests how the sickness response—seen as an emotional system—should also vary and transition from normal function to something that is considered to be "sick."

When trying to understand the traditional sensory systems (vision, hearing, feeling, smell, and taste), research has focused on factors such as reception (how a physical stimulus, such as light, sound, or pressure, is received and registered by a receptor), transduction (how the stimulation of the receptor is transmitted to a nerve signal), and coding (how characteristics of stimuli, such as lightness, loudness, or location in space, are represented in a signal that is understandable to the brain). This field of study is called sensory physiology. In study areas related to perception, the issues slowly slide over to more experiential factors where attention, subjective experiences, and interpretations are given more space. There, the focus has been on phenomena such as selection (how important stimuli are selected and reinforced at the expense of other information), organization (how parts of information are linked to a coherent whole and its effect on understanding), and interpretation (how we understand the things we perceive and what affects our views).

My argument is that, when it comes to understanding the inner world, one has relied too little on the perception psychology approach and ways of understanding how bodily and health-related signals are selected, organized, and interpreted. It should not replace the sensory bottom-up approach, but the perspectives must complement one another. The same goes for the emotional processes, which are closely linked to the perceptual ones. Both perceptual (external, exteroceptive) and interoceptive (inner) processes are natural starting points for emotional reactions, but it is also so that emotions control and influence how we understand both the outside world and our inner world. Not surprisingly, this works well for most people, but with a potential for dysregulation that can pose problems and contribute to ill health and functional variations. The similarities between emotional processes such as fear, sadness, and joy and the processes that control behavior when we are ill are striking, and we can again assume that evolution has contributed similar solutions to the similar tasks. It is likely that a variety of functional principles and "rules" apply to both common emotions and those arising from ill health.

What is an emotion?

To assist these diverse needs for regulating attention and behavior, there must be systems that prioritize and direct energy in desirable directions— systems that evaluate daily situations in relation to our goals. This is where emotions fulfill their important and immediate vital purpose. Overall, if the attainment of a goal moves further away, it gives rise to negative emotions, and if it comes closer, it creates positive emotions. These emotions arise to prepare us to act and to help us prioritize specific behaviors. The things we want to do, driven by the emotions, are perceived as urgent. In this way, emotions not only make us feel something, they also make us feel that we want to do something. Because of their ability to make us want to do something, one usually says that emotions have an imperative quality. This means that they can interrupt what we do and, so to speak, force themselves into our consciousness. But all this happens in a context in which emotions and their goals compete with other behaviors. They must therefore be regulated, and here we return to this important theme. Already in the nineteenth century, the classic American psychologist William James saw emotions as response tendencies that were malleable. We know this very well today, and emotional regulation is the subject of intense activity in treatment and research. As you have certainly noted, all this is once again an example of functional flexibility.

What are our most important, or what I will call "basic," emotions then?[1] One usually includes joy, sadness, fear, anger, and disgust; sometimes a

---

[1] The concept of basic and universal (consistent across cultures) emotions has been criticized in recent years. For the purpose of this chapter, discussing the emotions classically labelled as basic, and how they are understood, serves us well.

few more. Our emotions have been shaped during evolution and are to some extent inherited tendencies toward certain reactions. The emotions make us want to do what our distant ancestors had to do to pass on genes from one generation to the next, to quote psychology professor Arne Öhman. These basic emotions are thus quite similar across cultures. For many emotions there is also a similarity between species, which is why animal research has provided valuable knowledge for understanding the physiology and organization of emotions in the brain and the rest of the body. This is most obviously the case for fear, which is also the emotion we know most about.

Thus the emotions have a clear function, or rather several—they are behavioral tendencies with somewhat specific physiological foundations, which are generally (or at least have been) helpful in a number of prototypical situations. Joy arises in situations where we achieve goals, and this emotion aims to reinforce behaviors, increase cooperation, show affection, and make us continue on the course we began. They are thus rewarding, which makes us repeat behaviors. Grief or sadness arises in situations where we lose or remove ourselves from a goal, and has the function of getting us to seek help, change behaviors, and develop new plans. Anger occurs when something or someone prevents us from reaching a goal, and compels us to make a greater effort, assert our rights, or behave aggressively toward what it is that opposes the goal. Fear arises from threats to security or integrity, and functions to stop a behavior, to "freeze," to orient ourselves and read the surroundings, and to help us fight or flee. Finally, disgust arises in situations where we are at risk of being exposed to dirt, poisoning, or contamination, and has the function of helping us to reject or avoid the risk, vomit up unhealthy substances, or escape. The core emotions then lend themselves to other kinds of emotional reactions. For example, disgust lends itself to moral judgments, which by extension can be connected to situations where dirt, poisoning, or infection are relevant.

It is not far to go from feeling disgust to feeling sick, and onward to the body's total defense I previously described in terms of sickness response and our system to avoid infection. Herein lies a clear connection between the sickness response and our emotions. Before we analyze the sickness response and the experience of sickness as an emotion, I must make a further reflection. Emotions, according to the model I have presented, have traditionally been analyzed in terms of physiological changes that lay the groundwork for certain behaviors following the discovery and assessment of an urgent situation, together with an experience (Figure 7.1). One of the most important individuals in emotion research, the American Joe LeDoux, has recently criticized the traditional approach. He believes that much of emotion research has been guided by introspection in mental states that have a particular emotion attached to them, and therefore is

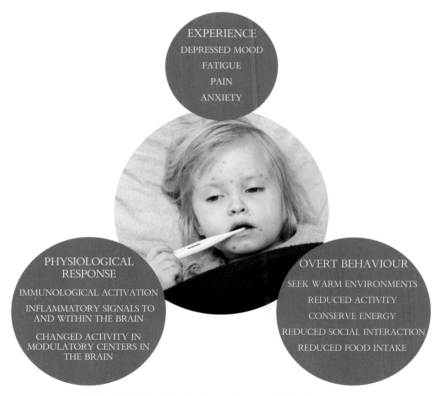

FIGURE 7.1 The body's physiological reaction to an infectious agent.
Mats Lekander and Rasmus Pettersson. Image: Shutterstock

governed by the language we use to describe these states. The basic phenomena we should understand instead, LeDoux argues, are the responses that occur when an organism detects and responds to important changes that are relevant to survival or continued well-being. He believes that this can be done to a great extent without linking them in a complicated way with confusing linguistic implications. LeDoux analyzes the emotions in terms of what he calls survival circuits, or as schematic reactions that occur when an organism perceives a danger to survival or continued well-being. Less emphasis is then placed on the words and language of emotions and more on the very function of survival. If the emotion occurs in systems that have the capacity for consciousness, conscious emotional feelings arise, but it is not necessary for the emotion to arise. The basic function is still there.

There is no doubt that handling micro-level threats from viruses or bacteria, which only white blood cells can detect, fits perfectly with this sort of survival system description. How these threats are discovered and addressed can thus be compared to the knowledge we have about both perception and emotion. The study of sick animals—which forms the fundamental basis of research on the disease response—is less associated with words related to emotions, which LeDoux argues have colored too much of how we have tried to understand the basic functions of traditional emotions. This is an extremely interesting area since our interpretation of an internal threat is influenced by expectations and linguistic structures, and thus is affected by how the threat is handled. How much should I let the feeling of wanting to be still control what I do when I have a temporary cold? Just as with other emotions, the intensity of our reaction and the extent to which it is linked to a behavioral response (should we act on the bodily feeling or simply continue what we were doing?) are influenced by previous experiences and knowledge. How dangerous is the pain or my fatigue, and does it represent a threat or not? Pain and fatigue, for example, can be interpreted as natural signals that do not threaten our health (the immune system is working fine and soon the fight against the invader will be over; the pain is due to exercise) or as signs of danger (my health is seriously threatened, and it is dangerous to move because it hurts).[2]

The interpretation we make and the value we assign to the signal in question depends on many factors. There are individual differences, where genetics and the environment make us react differently and cause us to interpret differently the physical and mental changes we experience. There are also cultural and historical differences that affect the interpretation of our symptoms. This can be done, for example, in accordance with society's values and the explanatory models that currently exist, something I will return to in Chapter 9 on social perspectives. All of these arguments about the sense of health and the conscious part of the sickness response are part of top-down processes, where interpretations and expectations affect the disease response itself, its intensity, and the behaviors that it affects.

Presented in this way, it is even more obvious that theories about how the brain manages threats are incomplete unless they include threats that arise or are detected within the body and that are to a great extent microscopically small. By connecting knowledge about the body's defense against microscopic threats to the long tradition of emotion research, a staggering opportunity arises: to better understand a central aspect of being human, namely how we perceive our health. In other words, threats to health activate survival systems that involve a number of changes in both our general physiology and in what we know, think, and do. And what we know, think, and do in turn affect physiological reactions and our health.

---

[2] The day before I submitted this manuscript, I lectured for almost a whole day to a group of very bright students, and we talked about the assessment of bodily health and when to stay home or not. In the middle of that discussion, I got a text message: "Dad, I feel really bad. Can I go home from school?" I read it out loud to the students, just as we were talking about such questions, together with my answer: "If you don't feel too bad and don't have fever, you don't need to be at home and can stay in school." I explained that my child is pretty good at noticing even minor bodily changes and that I had reason to believe that this was such an occasion. After a while, I got a new text message: "Dad, my teacher said I was allowed to go home." The students giggled a little and suggested that perhaps it was the *teacher* who was a little whiny. But when the lecture ended and the students had gone, I looked at the phone and read the following: "Dad, can you please hurry home? I just threw up."

Sickness is an emotion

Feeling sick is similar to both fear and disgust because avoidance is a strong component. These are defensive emotions. For fear, avoidance focuses on threatening stimuli or the situation in which they arise. Disgust makes us want to avoid a suspicious piece of food and thus guides our behavior to reduce the risk of poisoning. And the feeling of illness causes us to not only avoid further infectious stimuli, but indirectly also social interaction, food, and physical activity. Disgust arises, as just described, primarily from stimuli that can poison us or make us sick, but also constitutes (in the form of nausea, decreased appetite, and aversion to many foods) a natural part of feeling ill. A central brain area for disgust and such behavioral changes is the insula, which I have described as important in assessing bodily changes and which also responds to inflammatory activity.

From a larger perspective, we must consider the role of behavior and, by extension, the role of perceived health in relation to internal threats. Threats inside the body may (in the case of microbes like bacteria or viruses) or may not (in the case of cancer or injury) originate from the environment and come to pose a danger in the inner territory.

The more I study sickness behavior, the more similarities I find with what we usually call emotions. And all the more, I wonder why the flourishing academic literature about emotions does not involve the disease response. The chain of events that is triggered when a threat is detected at the microscopic level is analogous to what happens after major threats are detected by the naked eye. Threats at the micro level are not really identified until they are inside the body, but in most cases originate from the outside world. I also wonder why studies about our response to microscopic threats, that is, immunology and psychoneuroimmunology, seldom incorporate knowledge of how emotions contribute to our survival during life-threatening situations. It is likely that there are great functional similarities between various defense systems' approaches, and that one can therefore "borrow" and test principles across different branches of science. Behavior is a key component in our defense against both external and internal threats. It is obvious that genes that control behavior when we are threatened both from within and from the outside have been so important that they have spread and thrived throughout the course of evolution.

In fact, we only have one single integrated defense network, one that has emerged through gradual evolutionary adaptation. Each component of the network has been developed to fulfill specialized functions. We usually study these specialized functions individually without linking them on a central level. It is therefore time to take a more holistic approach to our understanding of human illness, including but not limited to behavior, which should be included as one of many levels of observation. In the long run we'll see renewed, modern healthcare that provides more efficient and thus cheaper interventions.

After all, emotions are highly preserved yet flexible schemes for organizing behavior to achieve certain goals in a way that served our ancestors well. This is very much the case even for the disgust response and the accompanying feeling of sickness. When we detect threats at the micro level, our response pattern matches the look of a "survival system" (the hard-core version of an emotion). But even from a slightly more traditional perspective, there are great similarities between what we usually mean by an emotion on one hand and a sickness response on the other.

Comparing the sickness response to other emotions

There are thus great similarities between micro-level threats and the way we respond to external threats, that is, through our traditional emotions. When researchers have tried to define what constitutes an emotion, some thought-provoking characteristics have emerged that were summarized by the researchers Paul Ekman and Richard Davidson. How these characteristics look and work differentiate the emotions from one another. If you analyze the sickness response from this perspective, you should learn something new at the same time as we test my idea about the disease response's compatibility with the other classic emotions. Let's wrestle a bit with the criteria formulated by Ekman and Davidson before we consider in Chapter 8 how malaise can be managed and perceived health improved.

The first typical feature is that the stimulus that triggers the emotion can be *detected and appraised automatically*. For external threats, we see this in a fear response that can be triggered without the involvement of the cerebral cortex in animals, or outside the consciousness of humans. And as far as infectious agents are concerned, we can in principle only perceive stimuli at the automatic level, through the "eyes" of the immune system, which I described in Chapter 5. Of course, the nervous system can also easily "suggest" the discovery of a contaminated substance. In such a case, we can falsely believe that we have been exposed to an infectious substance simply because we consider the risk of contamination to be high in a given situation. This belief can trigger avoidance behaviors and make us feel sick, or at least disgusted. The belief can set the stage for a small inflammatory reaction, which can happen through stress hormones. The same is true of external threats, which can be "suggested" by the nervous system so that the emotional response starts without the threat actually being present. Just imagine something you are afraid of at the same time as you touch your palms. Maybe you could feel that you were starting to sweat, which I myself just did when I triggered my discomfort for heights (even though I competed in ski-jumping when I was younger) by imaging that I was looking down from a high-rise building onto the street. As described in previous chapters, we are gifted with brains that are extremely skilled at suggesting the occurrence of numerous phenomena that might exist; in this way, the disease response differs very little from the classical emotions. This means that learned responses—such as a taste you associate with something that once nauseated you and still reminds you of the possible onset of stomach flu, or a careful scan of your body in search of symptoms—seem to be able to start at least parts of a sickness response. But the basic question is whether detection and assessment of triggering events occur at the automatic level, and it is obvious that this also fits well with the sickness response.

If emotions are general response patterns that have contributed to adaptation and the passage of genes, it is reasonable to assume that they are *triggered in response to similar events*. This is the second feature. Thus there should be common elements in the context in which emotions occur. At the same time, learning is important in influencing the exact nature of the stimuli that trigger the emotion, so that environmental information is used in conjunction with our systems for emotional reactions. We therefore have flexibility in how our ancestors' experiences are expressed in our daily lives. I have given several previous examples of how the context in which something occurs changes the intensity of a reaction. In terms of fear, it is clear that we have an innate reaction to sudden events, such as a loud noise, but the context determines whether the innate reaction (and often an initial reaction to "freeze") leads to fear and a behavioral response. Think back to the example of the Vietnam veteran who, after a loud noise, threw himself into a ditch instead of paying it minimal attention and ignoring it. Learning is a central part of this flexible adaptation to the environment, and it largely applies to both the immune system's and the usual emotional system's reactions.

The innate branch of the immune system responds by triggering a general inflammatory reaction when it recognizes a typical pattern of molecules it associates with danger. Therefore the sickness response is to a large extent a generalized response pattern that is triggered by similar events. At the same time, the force of the reaction can be regulated by a number of factors. The control systems that help to control the reactions (such as the stress hormone system) are set by events before or in connection with birth and early childhood. For acquired immunity, there is a very complex learning system that causes some white blood cells (lymphocytes) not to attack undamaged cells, but to respond to foreign or damaged cells. This process is established primarily during early childhood, but continues throughout the course of our lives, where we can, for example, become immune to the common cold virus we have encountered, or diseases we have been vaccinated against. The basic theme in this discussion of what constitutes an emotion is that similar events must precede the reaction, and here the sickness response compares well with traditional emotions.

A third feature of an emotion is that it should be *present in other primates*. This requirement is easy to check off. Although we cannot measure any subjective misery or self-rated health in other species, it is striking how the sickness response is basically the same in other mammals, not just primates, and humans. Biologically, the similarity is obvious, with the same or similar molecules that modulate physiological processes in a distinct way and that seem to reach similar targets in the brain. At the behavioral level, in both humans and animals, increased pain sensitivity, signs of fatigue, changes in sleep, signs of "depression" (such as the inability to enjoy things one normally appreciates), changes in motivation, appetite changes, and so on are seen—according to this criteria, there is no problem seeing the disease response as an emotion.

On the other hand, for the fourth feature (*quick onset*), and the fifth one (*brief duration*), it is more difficult and almost becomes a matter of definition. The features have to do with emotions controlling behavior, and should therefore be able to start quickly and then end quickly when the task is completed and the need no longer exists. If an inflammatory stimulus is injected into our bodies, we begin to feel sick after about an hour; this must be considered a slow response compared to the classic emotions. Similarly, it takes a couple of hours after such an injection for the response to subside. Although "short" and "long" are not defined in this context, the time duration of the sickness response hardly falls within the framework of "quick onset and short duration." On the other hand, the need is different here—for the sickness response, the goal is to save energy, reduce interest in social interactions, reduce appetite, reduce the risk of being exposed to external hazards while in a weakened state, and so on. The behavior and many physiological processes in the body are reorganized in a way that enhances recovery, but they need to last for a while after the threat is neutralized. Compare this with anger or joy, which can be more or less switched on and off in seconds or minutes. If we look at how behavior is used to avoid illness, as described in Chapter 5, it is different as compared to the sickness response. Avoidance behavior and suspicion can be triggered quickly to protect from contagion illness; this is largely done through disgust, but also through fear. In these cases, there is no doubt that the reactions can be quickly switched on or off, but it is not as obvious in terms of the sickness response. Once again, the mission is different: to be functional, the disease response needs to be extended. The time frame is thus a function of how the threat can be eliminated.

The sixth feature is *unbidden occurrence* of the emotion, so that it appears "uninvited." Here, the sickness response excels. The feeling of being sick appears like an unwanted guest, interrupting other activities. It asks for constant attention and reduces the capacity for other tasks, such as the ability to process information needed to meet other behavioral goals. For the sickness response, there is no qualitative research that describes how it manifests and how the experience develops over time. Can there be a typical development for how the disease response manifests? It would be unreasonable to assume that this must be the same for different people and on different occasions. In the absence of other data, I go to myself. Countless times I have felt a creeping discomfort in my body, a slight worry or anxiety without understanding why. It may take a while before it becomes so strong that it breaks into my consciousness, but when it does, I also know that it has been there for a while. Suddenly I stand there with a physical sense of worry paired with a feeling that what I am doing is less fun than usual. After a while, the explanation appears: a runny nose, bodily aches, and perhaps some symptom in my throat showing that it was "just" a cold. The experience of discomfort was not due to anything stupid I said or did, or to a gloomy forecast about the future. Rather, it was a reaction to a threat discovered at the micro level, wanting to "say something" to me so that I would change my behavior in an appropriate way. A close colleague, Martin Ingvar, tells a completely different story than mine: he feels somewhat elated and excited at the first sign of infection, before slipping into less pleasurable experiences. He suggests that the increased cortisol secretion that the immune response triggers (as part of regulating the strength of an inflammatory reaction) may be a reasonable explanation, as cortisol, in a sufficient dose, can certainly give rise to an exalted feeling. So it is quite possible. But since introspection is not an approved method for measuring hormone levels (although many, excluding my scholarly colleague, seem to think so when describing how much adrenaline they secreted during a particular task, or that they enjoy singing in a choir because it increased their endorphin levels), we must consider it as a working hypothesis. I think we can agree that the sickness response somehow manifests as an uninvited guest and asks for attention, but that we do not know what a typical course of events looks like.

One final reflection concerns the content of the message we receive from our bodies about a new condition. The intellectual level is not great—the body shouts "hello" and continues to draw our attention for a tediously long time. It's hard to silence these calls. But if one succeeds in ignoring the urge to keep still, and engages in something else that occupies our consciousness, it feels good to have escaped from the body's stubborn sickness messages for a while.

The seventh feature—a distinct physiological reaction that is related to the emotion (and which prepares the body for the behavior required)—can be addressed quickly. Here we have the well-known inflammatory response and its effects on other organs, such as the liver or the brain, with consequent behavioral changes, which I have described in previous chapters. The support for a distinct physiological reaction is in fact much stronger than for the classic emotions.

A last criterion is that an emotion should have a unique signal. The reason is that emotions do not elicit behavior in a vacuum. They clearly take place in a social context, and our emotions are used to understand others. It is of fundamental importance to be able to understand the feelings of others— to understand the needs of the unprotected child, to avoid betrayal and aggression, and to be able to reproduce. The brain even simulates the emotions of others in its own system for the same emotion. Our emotions are thus communicated to other people via cues and unique characteristics. For the classic emotions, there are external signs that a certain emotion is present in a certain human being, and there are also systems ready to read the available clues. The most obvious sign for humans is our facial expressions. They are also the best way to distinguish different emotional states in our peers. As organisms, we have a unique machinery for communicating through facial expressions, and with this we can make ourselves more clearly understood, influence others, and elicit compassion. When we talk, we take into account the facial expressions of others; a large part of our reaction to others' facial expressions is automatic and happens immediately, far away from the involvement of our consciousness. There is extensive and fascinating literature on this topic, but not for the sickness response. We simply do not know much about what it should look like, or if something in the signals differs from other emotions, and thus meets the criterion for being a unique signal. If we look at history and culture, we get some clues. In art, sick people usually look sad. The skin may be pale, posture is often poor, and the head is tilted forward. The similarity to depression is clear. A person whose attention is directed toward their body may be perceived as having an introverted gaze, but we do not know if this would simply correspond to a generally unfocused gaze or if there could be more direct clues about the shift in attention. There is little research on whether the sickness response is accompanied by a particular facial expression, but in Chapter 5 on the immunological defense system, I presented some features that appear to overlap with signs of fatigue and sadness. There I discussed different signs of illness in others, but this research is still in its infancy. For the sense of smell, there is some support for the notion that the cue is unique (at least in animals, and anecdotally in humans too), but less so for other sensory systems. When we deprive healthy people of sleep, we know that they look less attractive and more tired, and that others perceive their health as worse. But the people also look sadder, and the overlap with the emotion of sadness is obvious. In Chapter 5, I also mentioned how paleness in the face, droopy mouth corners, and hanging eyelids seemed to be linked to a recent inflammatory reaction—appropriately so, since contagiousness at that point may be considerable. But the ways in which health is apparent to others, and how these cues are perceived by others, is a relatively undeveloped field of research. Oddly enough, aren't signs of ill health, or perhaps just a changed general condition, important to discover in many healthcare professions?

In medicine, one speaks of the clinical eye, which is a metaphor for healthcare professionals being able to "see" the patient's condition, and I believe that more systematic research on signs of illness can help clinicians take another step on the path toward making good health assessments. But the growing body of research on how we avoid disease propels the field, together with research on placebos (which includes communication), which is why I expect more exciting future developments.

All in all, the sickness response is obviously quite similar to the classic emotions and holds its own when compared to Ekman and Davidson's criteria of what constitutes an emotion. If we adhere to LeDoux's hard-nosed approach (with highly regulated reactions when an organism perceives a danger to survival or well-being), we hardly even have to discuss the matter—the disease response is a missing puzzle piece that we must add so that it appears in its rightful context. A picture emerges in which internal threats are handled in ways that are similar to our systems for managing stimuli that arise during our interaction with the outside world.

But the main purpose is not to show that the sickness response is an emotion, but to learn about health and ill health by analyzing them from an emotional-psychological perspective. The benefits of this are huge. The long and successful tradition that exists in psychology and emotion psychology to understand and treat dysregulated emotional states can be borrowed to help us understand and influence health. In the same way that perception psychology can be utilized to also understand perception of inner states (interoception), emotion psychology can be leveraged to understand health and contribute to improved treatment. By applying a perspective of learning psychology, we have learned a lot since the 1970s about the sickness response and how it can be adjusted, and this has gradually developed into a cornerstone of placebo research. But an obvious benefit to applying an emotional-psychological perspective lies in the ability to understand how sickness responses are regulated; in other words, how neural and immune networks counteract and depress or reinforce disease symptoms based on context, interpretation, and other factors. Here we have a treasure chest ready to be opened. There are strong reasons to believe that the brain areas that are most important in controlling the intensity of classic emotions are also involved in regulating both our sickness response and our defense systems when trying to reduce the risk of becoming infected. Signs of this connection are being published both by my own research group and by colleagues around the world. This means that we will be able to better understand why we react so differently to illness, how we can harness these reactions, and why some people seem to have such a poorly functioning control system, which is central to their ill health. In Chapter 8, I'll discuss how we can influence subjective health factors.

Thus...

Emotion research has taken a huge step forward in recent decades by studying emotions from an interdisciplinary perspective. It has been taken for granted that researchers should use a combination of behavioral and physiological approaches to illuminate phenomena of interest. The approach has been successful not only in understanding general human behavior but also in understanding ill health, such as anxiety disorders, depression, ADHD, and borderline personality disorder. A large proportion of diffuse health problems that plague today's society can be better understood from a functional perspective that borrows thoughts and ideas from emotion research. Not least, new knowledge about emotional regulation can also help us understand how the sickness response, the stress response, and the health experience can be regulated. All of this is relevant to understanding individual symptoms of ill health, but is also relevant to understanding perceived health from a larger perspective. Since the way we experience our bodies and ourselves from a health perspective are largely affected by top-down processes, the question arises, how can you influence your own health experience? We will naturally take on this theme in Chapter 8.

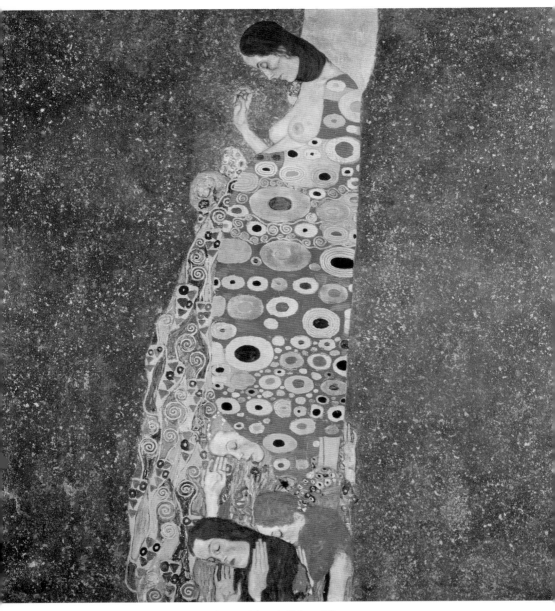

Gustav Klimt's "Hope II"

Bridgeman Images

8

CAN YOU AFFECT YOUR PERCEIVED HEALTH?

The answer to the question in the chapter title is simple: Yes. Just take a dose of endotoxin and you will soon view your health in a worse light. I find this idea strangely appealing, and hope to be able to redo my own endotoxin trial soon, preferably in the company of like-minded people. But all people do not belong in the category of "neuro nerds" like me, at least according to what one of my students claimed during a recent lecture. It is more natural to want to improve your health. But can you? The researcher in me answers dryly, "well, we don't know for sure," but my inner neuro nerd then comes to life and protests that we do indeed know for sure. "Show me the studies," says the researcher predictably and unimaginatively, but the neuro nerd answers with a long line of reasoning and series of arguments, triumphantly adding that studies with definitive answers are on their way. That is, of course, if one excludes studies in which self-rated health is worsened by injecting bacterial substances.

Hypochondriasis and health anxiety

I have previously described health anxiety, which includes unreasonable attention to bodily phenomena. The usual symptoms of health anxiety are misunderstanding bodily symptoms as signs of illness and being worried about being or becoming sick. An important part of health anxiety is maintaining the *possibility* of having or getting a disease. Another is to have an excessive fear of infections and becoming infected. There are several

The Inflamed Feeling. Mats Lekander, Oxford University Press. © Mats Lekander 2022.
DOI: 10.1093/oso/9780198863441.003.0008

diagnostic concepts that have to do with health anxiety and which, to complicate matters, change names now and then. In DSM-V, the latest edition of the diagnostic manual for psychiatric disorders, there is a new variant called *somatic symptom disorder*. In this diagnosis, you have significant focus on physical symptoms and worry excessively about these. Somatic symptom disorder is complemented by another new diagnosis, *illness anxiety disorder*, where the worry of having or getting a disease is more central than any symptoms. In this case, you have either no or very mild physical symptoms. The World Health Organization has an alternative diagnostic system called the ICD (International Classification of Diseases) in which hypochondriasis remains a diagnosis. In any event, the health anxiety component—anxiety about one's own health or the symptoms one experiences—is central to both.

Health anxiety seems to be common, especially among people seeking medical treatment, although there are no reliable calculations of the exact number. Using questionnaires, British researchers have estimated that this occurs in around 20 percent of people seeking medical care. In fact, early thoughts on hypochondriasis saw it as a male specialty, and one related to refinement and sensitivity. The additional costs within the healthcare system that can be attributed to hypochondriasis-like conditions are likely very large, and it is clear that many of these costs could be reduced if affected persons had access to effective treatment.

People suffering from health anxiety often suffer from a variety of symptoms. Let me present an illustrative case:

> A middle-aged, unemployed man with 10 children presents with headache, dizziness ("swimming of the head"), fatigue, chest pain, concerns about heart disease, mouth ulcers, heart palpitations, sleep problems, weakness, intermittent stomach pain, rashes and eczema, nausea, gastrointestinal problems and intermittent stomach pain, sea sickness, muscle spasms, colic, crying, anxiety, lethargy, small shaking attacks, a concern of imminent death, insomnia, tinnitus, tension in the chest, depression, visual disturbances, spasmodic nausea after meeting friends, exasperation, exhilaration with glowing sticks and dark clouds before his eyes, feelings of inertia, sharp shaking, feeling of general illness, boils, poor

resistance to infection, tooth and gum problems, nausea caused by emotion or stress, paleness, vomiting, twitches, miserable mood, dark and
gloomy thoughts, lethargy and stomach pain after too much sleep, and
bouts of rheumatism.

To clarify, I will add here that the man is not only the father of 10 children
but also of evolutionary biology. Yes, this is Charles Darwin. His condition was made worse by stress or, sadly, even by having fun. He wrote to a
person who wanted to meet him that he easily becomes mentally excited,
which always leads to spasmodic feelings of illness, and that he could not
endure a conversation with the person in question because he would appreciate it so much. It could serve as an excellent excuse. Admittedly, I find
symptoms of ill health to be quite interesting, but if a reader contacts me
and receives the answer Darwin gave, I hope that they notify my doctor.
Darwin, as I noted, got worse even from having a good time, and actually
experienced that he got significantly better from what I would describe as
the opposite of pleasure: a six-month cold-water treatment. Cold water
was supplemented with homeopathy, but Darwin was skeptical of the
latter treatment. It is likely that Charles Darwin in fact suffered from many
diseases[1] in the classic sense, but an excessive anxiety about his health is
also evident.

Another well-known person who suffered from severe health anxiety
was the Danish author H.C. Andersen. He wrote to his fiancée: "My friends
who know me so well, which is more than I do, say that my illness is imaginary; at least this imagination is a painful illness."[2] This description is apt,
except that it is not reasonable to simply call his state imagination. While
there may be some truth to the description—that is, that the problem lies
in the *interpretation* of the body and one's risk of ill health, and not in the

---

[1] A number of diagnoses have been suggested. One of these is hypochondriasis, another is
cyclic vomiting. The psychoanalytically influenced explanations of his illness state are more
imaginative, namely that it was due to distraught anger toward his father, and guilt over the
conflict with his former religious beliefs.

[2] Helweg HHC. *H.C. Andersen: En psykiatrisk studie*, 2nd ed. Köpenhamn: H Hagerups
Forlag; 1954.

body's condition itself—it does not capture the problem of health anxiety; instead it places the blame on the suffering person who has "actively" created the condition. If this is ignored, the last sentence ("this imagination is a painful illness") describes the core problem in health anxiety. If you take this seriously, you can easily imagine the suffering, and that the suffering can be perceived as irrational even by the victim. Receiving assurances about being healthy doesn't help. Here we can soon see how subjective health factors can be affected, and fortunately health anxiety is an area where we know quite a lot about what can make it better or worse. We'll start with things that make health anxiety worse, which we can then apply to our understanding of the things that can make us feel better.

"Noise" from the body is normal—noise that increases in certain situations, as the Canadian health anxiety researcher Gordon Asmundson has pointed out. This normal and harmless noise increases during stress, physical inactivity, and mild illness. In addition, it increases when we are doing something of particular interest in this book's perspective: checking our bodies for potential symptoms. Some people perceive harmless bodily changes as dangerous. Media reports on diseases, not surprisingly, increase health anxiety as well as the perceived risk of illness. Part of this has to do with coping strategies: repeatedly ensuring one's condition increases focus on the body. "Doctor shopping" to get a third, fourth, or fifth reassuring opinion thus has a price.

The American researcher Bunmi Olatunji has shown that both the symptoms of health anxiety and the tendency to feel disgust can be increased in healthy people if they devote themselves for a week to checking their health more than they usually do. These behaviors included, for example, checking lymph nodes, weighing themselves, measuring body temperature, taking their heart rate, or looking for blood in the urine. At the end of the week, symptoms of health anxiety had increased, as well as the number of potentially infectious objects they avoided. I have described distaste as an important part of health anxiety and as something that is related not only to *being* sick, but also to *avoiding* illness. Distaste drives avoidance behaviors. True, people with health anxiety are more likely than others to feel distaste. This tendency to feel distaste, or disgust, is usually considered a stable personality trait, but Olatunji also tested if it changed. Indeed, the participants who increased their health-checking behaviors also increased their propensity for distaste, especially the kind that has to do with avoidance of contamination.

In addition to the suffering associated with health anxiety, it is strongly linked to sick leave—probably surprising to no one. Health anxiety is also commonly associated with conditions such as depression and other anxiety disorders.

The question then is whether it is possible to successfully treat health anxiety, and the answer is yes. Under the leadership of the researcher and psychologist Erik Hedman, we have shown, in a series of studies, that health anxiety can be very effectively treated with cognitive behavior therapy. This can be performed as a regular face-to-face treatment, over the internet, or even by carefully following the instructions in a book. The efficacy is great, and the intervention goes something like this: do the same things as in the study described above in which disgust and health anxiety were increased in healthy people—but in the opposite way. In other words, gradually expose yourself to what you are afraid of. The anxiety will decrease significantly.

The concept is the same as with other anxiety problems, where a specific phobia is the simplest example: if you are afraid of spiders, you approach spiders in a well-organized and safe way in order to make the nervous system relearn. Practical experience, carried out in a way that has been developed within a scientific framework, is what is needed to reduce anxiety. In this case, one may be exposed to events or situations that cause health anxiety. It can involve physical exertion and even reading about things that can make you sick or die. It can also involve daring to touch an object that you think is disgusting. Since anxiety is maintained both by avoiding such events and situations and by performing controlled behaviors when exposed to them, an important component is added after exposure. This is called response prevention and is based on the fact that you do not, for example, wash your hands when you touch what you do not want to touch, or that you do not check your heart rate after physical exercise. This means that in response to the discomfort you feel during the exposure, you should not escape the situation, or call a doctor, if that is what you usually do. In short, this type of 12-week treatment reduces health anxiety significantly for most people.

Had I been Darwin (and please note that I would agree to a swap if it comes into question), I would have preferred 12 weeks of treatment delivered via a computer (remember that not even Darwin knew about electromagnetic hypersensitivity at that time) to six months of cold-water treatment.[3] And also gotten well. Perhaps I would miss the symptoms as a topic of conversation. To quote H.C. Andersen: "If I am not allowed to talk about my pains, they don't do me any good."

Health anxiety is basically sound because there are good reasons to worry about getting sick when standing in front of a person spreading microorganisms through a cough, and it may be wise to wash your hands after they've being in a creepy place, or change your behavior when your body rebels and shouts that you are sick. Thus the tendency can reasonably be seen as positive and protective. The problem, however, the tendency to become overly sensitive to signs of illness and when the anxiety becomes disproportionately high.

If people with health anxiety easily become both disgusted and worried, it is reasonable for them to respond "effectively" when they pick up signs of illness from their surroundings—and maybe their reaction is simply too effective. We have tested this by showing pictures of ill people to individuals with health anxiety (see Figure 8.1). The people in the pictures look more or less sick, and some cough and are obviously ill. We have taken advantage of the opportunity to explore these questions when treating patients over the internet who are sitting in front of a computer, and we have compared their responses to those of

---

[3] Tragically, Darwin's daughter Annie died after a month of treatment at the clinic Darwin visited. In addition to water treatment (hydrotherapy), the treatment package included clairvoyance, mesmerism (a kind of hypnosis), and, as I said, homeopathy.

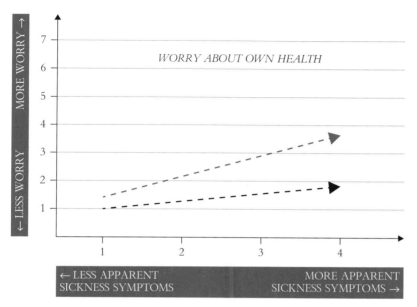

FIGURE 8.1 People with health anxiety are afraid of being or becoming sick, and their bodily signals are signs that they have serious illnesses. We have investigated whether the fear of getting sick also causes them to overestimate signs of illness in others by showing them photos of faces that look healthy or sick. The figure shows that the sicker a person in a photo appears to be (1 = no apparent signs of illness, 4 = strong apparent signs of illness), the more health anxiety patients' worry about their own health increases (red dotted line) compared with people without health anxiety.

control subjects with varying degrees of health anxiety who fall below the threshold for the diagnostic criteria. In this study we found that the stronger the participant's health anxiety, the more anxious and disgusted they felt when seeing the pictures, and the more they worried about their own health. The more disease symptoms the individuals in the pictures displayed, the more the severity of the symptoms were over-interpreted by the health anxiety patients compared to the control subjects. The subjects with health anxiety perceived the people in the pictures as sicker, more contagious, and less attractive to spend time with. No wonder that health anxiety leads to problems with social situations and avoidance. Since health anxiety is characterized by symptoms and concerns about health in the absence of objective diagnoses, I think that health anxiety is a particularly interesting branch within the subjective health field. I shall soon return to this topic.

Perceived health varies over time

Because self-rated health (how individuals say they perceive their general state of health) is such a good predictor of future death and other objective measures of ill health, one might think that it is not possible to affect it very much. I touched on this question in Chapter 6 on the general state of health and described how the assessment was affected by activating the immune system or by shortening sleep time to just a few hours a night.

Pain, fatigue, positive and negative emotional states, and inflammation are things that most people are affected by when they appraise their general state of health. These conditions are hardly stable. Their functions involve, after all, in making us change our behavior: you have to suffer from pain so that you want to stay still and not repeat what caused the misery, feel tired so that you want to rest and sleep, or feel happy (or sad) so that you want to continue (or discontinue) what you are doing.

Changes in living conditions should therefore influence not only your health experience "now," but also your general health assessment. Stress appears to increase health anxiety. Could it have a similar effect on one's assessment of our general state of health? During Karolinska Institutet's medical education program, there is an extensive exam that covers the first and more theoretical parts of the education that students take before beginning the clinical training; that is, before they start working with patients. Wisely, one must pass the exam in order to continue with the clinical education. Of course, the students get very stressed. And then I mean REALLY STRESSED. Nevertheless, for one study we did, they were able to fill in questionnaires, give blood samples, urinate in bottles each morning for urine tests, and blow in various contraptions to measure lung function. As a comparison, we measured the same elements during a calmer study period without an approaching exam, when much lower stress estimates were made. To be on the safe side, we even performed some measurements in the reverse order, during different years, and in connection with a similarly demanding exam (pathology) during another part of the year. The students' self-rated general health deteriorated significantly during the stressed periods compared to the calm ones. Remember that we are talking here about hefty assignments with weeks of intensive preparation required to pass the exam.[4] So stress seems to be able to affect self-rated health, even though little research is available on the topic.[5]

As I described earlier, we have good reason to believe that self-rated health is made worse by paying attention to symptoms, scanning the body, and checking our health status too often. In a large study, we were given an unforeseen opportunity to study this effect, since the question of self-rated health (framed as health "for the day") was inadvertently included twice in the same questionnaire—once before and once after a number of symptom questions in which respondents were asked to answer if they had suffered from a number of symptoms during the day. The list of symptoms was almost at the Darwinian level, with 22 suggestions of bodily or mental phenomena to consider. So when the health question appeared a second time, after pondering whether they had experienced any symptoms that day, people on average answered that their health was worse than before—despite the fact that they had answered the exact same question just a few minutes before. The more symptoms people estimated they had during the day, the greater the deterioration in the second question. The difference was small, but since we had many participants, we could still see a statistically significant difference and be sure that their assessment had indeed changed.

---

[4] It is wise to remember that, in most cases, the students could hardly have done better on the exam without a stress response, but probably worse. Worrying generally leads to preparation, thereby allocating energy to what is important. But we know from experience that the discomfort and anxiety can also be so great that it becomes an obstacle. Many students stated that the stress was so great that their performance was negatively affected.

[5] These research results have not been published and are thus not peer reviewed, as they were removed from the journal we published our general results in, as the journal's editors did not view their significance in the same way we did.

One can explain such an effect on several complementary levels. One explanation may be more neuroscientific, where we can assume that we activate the parts of the brain that deal with interoception; imagining symptoms that you may to some extent have also activates the brain areas that are involved when you experience something in reality. When attention is directed toward the body, it is then possible to detect, amplify, or even create symptoms (like nocebo), which then affect how you appraise your health. This is a bit like the "medical student sickness" where students in med school find themselves experiencing the very symptoms associated with the disease they are studying—I might add from personal experience that this also works well during psychology studies.

I once lectured with the therapist Åsa Nilsonne, who directly, before my eyes, manipulated how many of the students experienced pain at a certain moment. She did this by asking them to sit quietly and reflect on their bodies for a minute. After the minute was over, a fairly large number of students reported pain when asked, although only a few did when asked before the exercise began. The students were then asked to tell the student next to them about a personally engaging and positive experience, to make it lively, and to immerse themselves in the other person's story when listening. After that, the pain question was raised again—but now not a single student reported feeling any! Needless to say, chronic pain disorders are neither invented nor under the suffering person's control, and can involve a problem in how pain is regulated.

A more cognitive explanation of the phenomenon than the one dealing with attention, interoceptive processes, and nocebo, is about *availability bias* (or *anchoring bias*, a concept with a partially overlapping meaning). Anyone who has read Daniel Kahneman's book *Thinking, fast and slow* knows what I'm talking about. The phenomenon is about the fact that something that is more available, recent, or easy to think about when making an assessment is given greater importance and influences your judgment. I previously described an example of how one's assessment of the climate might be affected by the weather on the day the assessment is made, which can be explained by the weather being available and relevant on that particular day and thus given greater importance, compared to how the weather generally (that is, the climate) is judged to be. Married couples who are asked how often they take care of household chores substantially overestimate their own efforts. It is easy to remember occasions when you have done your own chores, but it is difficult to remember when you have not done so, which is a result of accessibility bias (so a tip in private life is to watch one's tendency to overestimate one's own contributions to the household). A final example concerns Kahneman's and Tversky's experiments where they let people estimate the product of the numbers $1 \times 2 \times 3 \times 4 \times 5 \times 6 \times 7 \times 8$ within five seconds. The median response was 512. For participants who instead had to estimate the product of $8 \times 7 \times 6 \times 5 \times 4 \times 3 \times 2 \times 1$, the median response was 2,250. That the correct answer is 40,320 is not relevant here, but rather the fact that the first numbers are given greater importance in the assessment via anchoring bias.

So when you have just thought of a moment during the day when you had a headache, you then make the assessment that this was a typical condition for the day, which makes you evaluate your current health as worse. Similarly, when you are asked about your health, a search process starts, which is interrupted when enough information has been produced, and a *prototypical* situation (that is, a situation that is perceived as typical) is created in your memory. The information that is easily accessible has a greater influence on your judgment than other alternatives due to availability bias. The condition that is presented is perceived as typical and thus representative of one's general health.

The role of mindset

As mentioned, the appraisal of a threat affects how strong the stress response becomes. It has long been known that factors such as judgment, perceived control, social support, and so on are part of the stress equation. We should therefore be able to influence the context in which something is presented and thereby affect both the subjective experience and objective measures of bodily change. The reasoning is clearly reminiscent of placebo and is roughly the same phenomenon. American researcher Alia Crum examined whether *attitudes* toward the physical act of cleaning affected the cleaning experience and whether biological aspects were affected. The cleaning women were given examples of how their work corresponded to official physical activity guidelines. Physical activity is good, isn't it? The researchers found that, compared to cleaners who did not receive this information, the women felt that they got more physical activity than before, even though their actual behavior did not change. In addition, they lost weight and had lower blood pressure, less body fat, reduced waist-hip ratio, and lower BMI! In another study, Crum reported how the secretion of a hunger hormone was affected by whether research subjects believed that a milk shake they drank had a very high energy content and that they "allowed themselves" to drink it, or if exactly the same drink was presented as a low-calorie drink (which in fact it was). If the participants thought that the milk shake had a higher energy content than it actually had, the secretion of the hunger hormone ghrelin was affected. This hunger hormone clearly increased before the shake was consumed and was then switched off among those who thought they were consuming something good but less healthy.

I would like to see studies with such spectacular results replicated by other researchers, but it is nevertheless interesting to note that Crum and colleagues have done similar studies in which the approach to stress as either helpful or dangerous affects one's response to certain stressors. Epidemiological studies that looked at the relationship between severe stress and future health found that both stress itself and the *perception that stress is dangerous* are associated with poorer health development. The perception that stress is dangerous may thus be a risk factor in itself. We shall return to this perspective in Chapter 10.

"No news is good news," and good health is quiet, as I mentioned earlier. But what if it is *not* quiet because we are prompted by health messages and frightening images to evaluate our health too often, and have high expectations for what life should be like, at the same time as we are living longer with chronic diseases? If we identify something that could be better, it activates negative emotions, as I have described, whose function is to help us reach our goals by changing behaviors. If we pay attention to the body by constantly evaluating our health, we may:

1. Discover symptoms we were previously unaware of,
2. Activate negative emotions, even in cases when symptoms do not signal ill health but are a part of life, and
3. Judge our health as being worse than previously thought.

If we judge our health to be poorer, are we at greater risk of ill health? It is far from certain that negative health assessments actually cause ill health, but it cannot be ruled out. If we worry and are dissatisfied, it can affect health behaviors (such as sleep, diet, exercise, following medical advice). If nothing else, we feel worse, which can be bad enough. So the cost of focusing too much on one's own health is that we are activating bodily circuits that should only be activated when something is wrong, and which when activated are likely to have unnecessarily negative consequences.

Healing thoughts?

Positive psychology has swept across the world with its message of focusing on factors that make life better rather than focusing on problems and dysfunctions. It has been a much-needed response to the strong focus that research, and most healthcare, has had on negative factors. At this level, it's hard to contradict.

It has been easier to study factors that affect us negatively than those that protect us in the long run. And it has been extremely difficult to organize preventive care so that we maintain health rather than trying to return to better health once we are ill. But with this positive psychology trend—even though well-needed—a wave of self-help prophets with bestselling products have often not followed scientific advice or common sense.[6] With this come statements that make everything seem so simple: "Don't ruminate—turn off the negative thinking" or "Stop being morose—put away your sorrows and soon the sun will shine again," to paraphrase popular authors and lecturers.

How much does this help? Can I hear a bad conscience raise its voice? An important point here is that the ability to feel good and experience happiness is admittedly not just a trait you happen to have, or a reaction that you passively experience, but in fact is also a skill. In other words, the ability to appreciate things that should be appreciated can in part be learned. For example, you can try to get in the habit of pausing, helping others, or being present in the moment when something good happens, and so on. This is part of meditation and mindfulness training and, I would argue, part of raising children (that is, helping them learn to seize the opportunity to enjoy life and be in the moment when opportunity presents itself).

But how much does jaunty advice help the millions of people who suffer from anxiety or depression? Importantly, with today's health trends, much responsibility is placed on the individual. With this perspective, we tend to ignore problems related to societal structures and blame ourselves for failing or for feeling ill. Conditions and demands may be overwhelming and unhealthy, and when possible should be changed rather than merely coped with. A condition like depression needs treatment and it is hard to think one's way out of it.

A problem with the application of positive psychology is that, in many cases, you draw hasty conclusions. For example, we know that there is a certain relationship between the amount of positive emotions one expresses and life expectancy, but that does not justify advising people to "turn that frown upside down." It sounds obvious but is worth pointing out that quick unfounded advice on health and lifestyle is common. For

---

[6] Please note that self-help can be very helpful, as when you, on your own, go through a treatment which is well tested and based on scientific studies.

me, it is reminiscent of the societal trends of the 1980s when many cancer patients I met as a doctoral student had read bestselling books about "exceptional cancer patients" who "managed" to fight against and even think away tumors. It is fatal to take hope from a person, but is it not worse to give false hope? So if I fail to be exceptional, do I have to blame myself if the cancer spreads? I read some of those books with one thought ringing loudly in my head: those poor patients.

Psychological treatments and perceived health

Subjective suffering is central to mental ill health. While this is certainly an understatement, there are conditions in which suffering is not at all related to the degree of illness, is denied, or conversely, is even accompanied by good mood, in some extreme examples. While in recent years the pharmaceutical industry has had difficulty producing new drugs for mental ill health, brick by brick psychological treatment has added to the construction of a small castle of evidence-based treatments. For psychological diagnoses such as depression, anxiety disorders (a variety of conditions), and *insomnia* (difficulties falling asleep or maintaining sleep, impairing daytime functioning), there is effective psychological treatment. These treatments are often recommended as first-choice options, with better long-term efficacy than the drugs typically prescribed for the corresponding conditions. The negative side effects are also weaker. In addition to measures of depression, anxiety, and sleep disorders, the subjective symptoms described in this book (including worry, low mood, and fatigue) can also be reduced. Behavioral treatment for chronic pain reduces the suffering and disability associated with underlying conditions, although not always the intensity of the pain. The degree of disability thus decreases to some degree for most people.

One can thus say that illnesses with subjective characteristics and their most common symptoms can be addressed through psychological treatment. Cognitive behavioral therapy is the treatment form with the strongest support, although it is not the only one that has been shown to be effective.

As mentioned, individuals with health anxiety are greatly helped by cognitive behavioral therapy. One can thus say that subjective health is indirectly improved in people with health anxiety because, by definition, they feel ill despite lacking a diagnosis before starting treatment, and then get much better. But what about the holy grail of subjective health measures, self-rated health, formulated as a single small but powerful question on one's general state of health? Here we have the reason why the researcher in me was critical of the "neuro nerd" at the beginning of the chapter: because we and others have only begun to publish our attempts to influence this measure in optimized treatments. The best way is to randomize people into different treatments and then compare the results of the treatment you are interested in with those of the group that received a control treatment or no treatment at all. Some of these studies have now been published and have shown positive results. After treatment, health anxiety patients appraised their health as clearly better than they did before treatment, while untreated patients did not improve in this way. Feelings of sickness decreased in parallel. We also saw corresponding improvements in people being treated for chronic stress. In a study of psychological treatment for pain patients, we also studied self-rated health before and after treatment. Patients receive some help from this treatment—not to eliminate the pain, but to increase functioning and live a life closer to their values, despite the pain.[7] We compared two treatments, and the one that showed the fastest effect also showed significantly better self-rated health compared to the other group. Six months after treatment, the second treatment group (which received an active relaxation intervention) had caught up to the first and both had now significantly improved compared to their status before starting treatment. The control group was not untreated here, and it is important to remember that we could not

---

[7] The treatment is called ACT—acceptance and commitment therapy—and is a variant of cognitive behavioral therapy.

compare the treatment results with those of patients who did not receive any treatment at all, which could indicate the course of natural recovery, or how the condition would typically develop over time when untreated.

Top-down processes and health

I have pointed out that top-down processes (where expectations, prior knowledge, or "rules" affect a signal that enters the brain) are important not only for understanding the world around us but also for the world that exists within us. I have argued that these "hypothesis-driven" processes that meet the flow of information from the body are less explored than when they come from the external world, and its scientific history is shorter. But they need to be studied and understood as they are central to human health, and should be central to how health is promoted and ill health is treated and prevented.

As a reader, you have now noticed many examples of how the body and its condition can be described as a hypothesis that the brain has, that this hypothesis changes depending on the circumstance, and that it can be affected in different ways. You have learned about placebos, immune system conditioning, and several other phenomena. In this chapter you have read numerous examples related to health anxiety that teach us how our subjective health is related to our behaviors, and how the mere fact that we think about symptoms can make us judge our general state of health to be worse than it really is. All are clear examples of how malleable health is even after bodily messages have reached the brain.

One poorly understood area is how the regulation of bodily phenomena differs from person to person. It may be that not all people have the same ability to regulate activity in parts of the brain that deal with the interoceptive processes described in Chapter 2. Brains obviously differ among people, and certain parts are larger in some brains and smaller in others. The primary area for receiving and processing information from the body, the insula, is one area that is significantly different among different people.

A reasonable hypothesis is that this relates to how intensely we react to a physical change. Similarly, the orbitofrontal cortex in the frontal lobes differs greatly among people in its construction, and findings indicate that this is related to different functioning. Studies of people with the chronic pain condition fibromyalgia have relatively smaller volume in another part of the frontal lobe, the anterior cingulum. Moreover, the longer the people had suffered from chronic pain, the larger the difference between this group and other people seemed to be. Both of these areas (the orbitofrontal cortex and anterior cingulum) are central to regulating emotions and bodily signals. They, along with some other areas in the frontal lobes, are directly involved in top-down processing of signals from the body.

When asking people to increase their control over an emotionally engaging stimulus, let's say an unpleasant image, the person may view the image as though it comes from a movie recording, that the unpleasant scene is quite distant from them, or a similar strategy. This strategy can be called cognitive control or cognitive reinterpretation. Another term that means almost the same thing is emotional regulation. When people use this type of control—like when I interpreted my body's signals as signs of exercise rather than stress while running to the train—they recruit their frontal lobes (including the orbitofrontal cortex) and reduce the discomfort they would otherwise feel. Emotional regulation is a "skill," and people's skill levels differ. It is evident in conditions such as borderline personality disorder, which is characterized by rapid and emotional oscillations that are hard to control. It is obvious that we as individuals are not equally good at exercising control over our emotions during different times in life. A prime example of this is after sleep deprivation—we may suddenly say things we thought would never cross our lips, or phrase comments in an unnecessarily blunt way. For my own part, I have seen that my parenting ability is at a low when I sleep too little, and I can sometimes hear my inner voice protest against my own behavior—a clear lack of control. Perhaps the connectivity between the frontal lobes and the deeper parts of the brain involved in emotional reactions decreases due to sleep deprivation. This may be a mechanism behind lack of emotional control after a short sleep. A somewhat surprising effect of top-down processes for those with sleep issues is that people with insomnia underestimate their length of sleep. In fact, insomniacs tend to think that they are awake during periods of sleep. Providing them with information on how much they sleep has been shown to reduce fatigue, worry, and negative thoughts. Daytime functioning is thus improved by this information. Consequently, addressing insomniacs' underestimation of their sleep time is part of their cognitive behavioral therapy. Although sleep length has only been shown to increase by about 20 minutes after treatment—a good but modest change—it nevertheless resulted in reduced fatigue and a steady improvement in their perceived daytime function.

You can try to change your thoughts and attitudes, and manage your sleep and general health as well as you can to control your emotions. This is not bad, but we don't know for sure if we have really changed the brain's activity or the connection between different brain areas in the way we think. We cannot spontaneously know how much activity is happening in a particular part of the brain because we do not have receptors that report activity to other brain areas that are capable of compiling it and helping us understand what is happening. But imagine if one could measure activity with neuroimaging and monitor it in a test subject while they were in the scanner, and in this way *teach* them to increase activity in a brain area that controls emotions. This would be top-down control, if anything. This principle is called neurofeedback and has actually been tested for a number of years. "Interesting and possibly promising" is how I would summarize the results. For example, one review shows that a little over half of the studies done on psychiatric conditions have shown statistically significant improvements. But for a number of reasons, there is a long way to go until it can be considered reasonably efficient. So decide for yourself about the technique you will spontaneously use to control your emotions when needed, and use it instead of looking for a brain-imaging therapist (a specialty that, to my knowledge, does not actually exist).

The top-down processes are thus deeply involved in our health—those that are objectively measurable and the subjective ones best measured through careful, well-validated questions and interviews, and behavioral measures. Research on the regulation of emotions is rapidly increasing, but so far it is primarily focused on some of the classic emotions, like fear, and less on phenomena that are more obviously physical or related to self-awareness. This is where fatigue, stress, pain, distaste, shame, and the feeling of illness come into the picture. We believe, and have some evidence, that the anterior cingulum is involved in these processes, together with the anterior insula, parts of the frontal lobes such as the orbitofrontal cortex, and what is called the dorsolateral prefrontal cortex. The orbitofrontal cortex has an interesting role not only because it participates directly in the inhibition of emotional responses, but also because it seems to provide a "green light" to refrain from monitoring internal or external events, or to trigger a behavior in response to them. This type of function is about signalling well-being and sending a "comfort signal." In other words, if conditions are good, there is no need to act.

Interestingly, the orbitofrontal cortex receives signals not only from the classic sensory systems (taste, smell, touch, sight, and hearing) but also from visceral (interoceptive) systems. This means that the area can monitor both the outer and inner worlds, assess comfort and discomfort along with expectations and goals, and contribute to decisions about possible behavioral changes.

Psychological treatment often includes techniques to harness top-down processes of the inner world. It thus involves interoceptive processes that include the insula and parts of the frontal lobes. We have already discussed the treatment of health anxiety. Another example is the treatment of pain, in which the fear of pain and of movement (kinesiophobia) may have become an equally large problem as the pain itself. One task for the therapist is to reduce the sense of danger patients associate with pain and movement, so that needed and valued behaviors can more easily take place. The therapist helps the patient to direct behaviors toward reaching overarching and important long-term rather than short-term goals and rewards, so that brain systems can learn about and thus evaluate the pain signal differently. In panic disorder, there is a great fear of the body's reactions, such as heart palpitations and altered breathing. One successful treatment is to reduce the fear by letting the person experience that the symptoms are not dangerous—if the symptoms are allowed to "spike" and the patient's normal tendency to flee from the situation is suppressed, the system learns that the symptoms are not dangerous and do not need to be followed by certain behaviors, such as avoidance. Top-down processes can thus be trained through psychological treatment.

It is reasonable that a certain level of attention is advantageous, but some people care too much *or too little* about internal signals. For example, in prolonged stress, it is thought that, for some individuals, the inability to listen to the body in itself contributed to the development of exhaustion. This is believed to have led to too little recovery. But it is unclear how far training in top-down processes can go. Probably not to the extreme level of what was called "La belle indifférence"—a lack of concern toward one's symptoms. All in all, it seems clear, however, that a poor ability to evaluate one's symptoms can mean that a person does not sufficiently notice or care about bodily signals. This perspective fits well with the great similarities in sickness response across species described in Chapter 4, and with the idea that a certain degree of health anxiety is advantageous if we are to remain healthy. Evolutionary pressure to involve behavior in our disease defense arsenal has obviously been great; ignoring bodily signals to rest would have reduced the chance of survival.

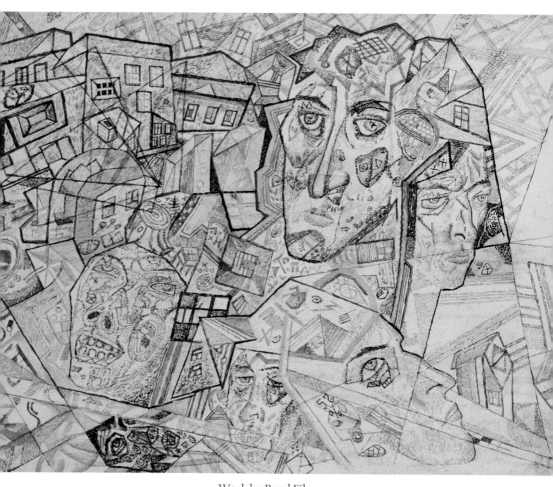

Work by Pavel Filonov

9

HOW SOCIETY AFFECTS OUR HEALTH

If health involves such strong subjective elements created by the brain in collaboration with the immune system, among others, it must also be a general social issue of great relevance beyond what we associate with standard healthcare. The view of health affects objective and perceived health in several ways. Where the boundary is drawn between normal and sick, at certain moments, has consequences for care and for individuals' right to compensation from the insurance systems. How health is explained and how ill health is described in society affects how the brain interprets symptoms, how people experience them, and thus how they are presented to healthcare providers. Another societal aspect, as I have shown before, is that openness toward foreign people, and disapproval of norm-violating behaviors, is affected by both actual and perceived health risks. In addition, health is a *lifestyle* that is closely related to consumption, which may push citizens to search for signs of illness. But how do we take subjective symptoms seriously—since they are so strongly linked to harsh outcome measures that no one can ignore—without making matters worse by encouraging people to fixate more on their health and on how they experience their bodies?

Health through the distorted mirror of society

A mirror reflects light but also shapes the images we see. Society and culture are effective mirrors through which we can judge whether we

The Inflamed Feeling. Mats Lekander, Oxford University Press. © Mats Lekander 2022.
DOI: 10.1093/oso/9780198863441.003.0009

are healthy or ill. In the book *Magic mountain,* Thomas Mann describes life and culture as it happened in a sanatorium in Switzerland. There, patients suffering from lung disease gather to breathe mountain air and recover from tuberculosis. The main character Hans Castorp comes to the luxurious sanatorium Berghof in Davos to visit his cousin Joachim, looking forward to what he thinks will be three restful holiday weeks. After discovering that Castorp is also ill and in need of treatment, the stay is extended from three weeks to seven years. The book describes a sanatorium culture that can make the healthiest of characters feel sick. At breakfast and dinner, fever and other symptoms are discussed. Two powerful weapons are used as antidotes to the disease: rest cures in balcony deck chairs and psychoanalysis. Treatments take place while resting on thick bolsters under camel-hair blankets on sanatorium balconies in recliners next to the snow-covered balcony parapets looking out over the nearby mountains (see Figure 9.1). A few books, something to drink, rest, and the opportunity to really think

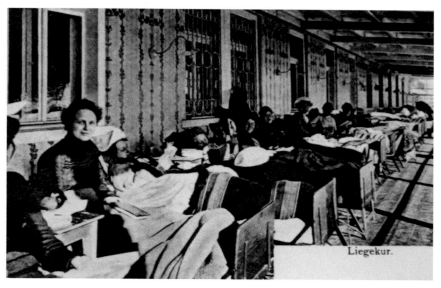

FIGURE 9.1 Patients treated with "rest cure" at a Davos sanatorium in the late 1800s.

and feel. Who wants to be healthy in such circumstances? And per-haps more importantly, who *can* be healthy in such circumstances? Psychoanalysis helps with the need for introspective exercises—of doubtful benefit to those with tuberculosis. The psychoanalyst Dr Krokowski "dissects the souls" of the patients, questioning whether Hans Castorp really is, as he claims, perfectly healthy: "But then you are a phenomenon well worth studying! I have never met a perfectly healthy person!"

Upon closer examination, and despite his assurances, Hans Castorp is in fact not completely healthy, and he is drawn into the sanatorium's routines and a world in which diseases and its symptoms play a central role. Triumphantly, he buys his first beautifully dec-orated fever thermometer, and with even greater triumph he even-tually reports a temperature of 37.6°C. He thus qualifies as being among the truly sick: those who have a fever. Entering the world of disease, he stops winding up his pocket watch and loses his grip on time and space.

The book was long unpublished, but when finally released, Thomas Mann described reality's equivalence to the beginning of the novel. He had visited his wife, who was staying at a sanatorium (see Figure 9.2) for treatment.

> I had been at the so-called Berghof ten days, sitting out on the balcony in cold, damp weather, when I got a troublesome bronchial cold. Two specialists were in the house, the head physician and his assistant, so I took the obvious course of consulting them.
>
> I accompanied my wife to the office, she having been summoned to one of her regular examinations. The head doctor "/.../", thumped me about and straightway discovered a so-called moist spot on my lung.
>
> If I had been Hans Castorp, the discovery might have charged the whole course of my life. The physician assured me that I should be acting wisely to remain there for six months and take the cure.[1]

---

[1] Mann T. The magic mountain. London: Secker & Warburg; 1924.

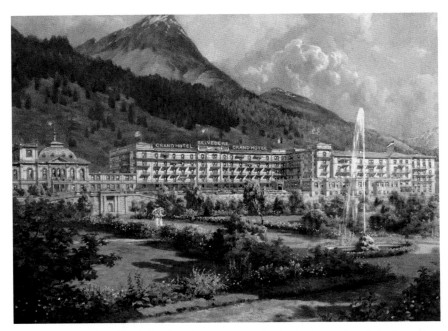

FIGURE 9.2 Grand Hotel Belvédère in Davos. A classic Davos hotel, built in 1875, that hosted Thomas Mann.

Thomas Mann declined to stay, wrote his novel instead, and was, "despite" this,[2] awarded the Nobel Prize in Literature in 1929. A passage in the book reads as follows:

> The conversation at table was not lively. Joachim talked politely with Frau Stohr, inquired after her condition and heard with proper solicitude that it was unsatisfactory. She complained of relaxation. "I feel so relaxed," she said with a drawl and an underbred, affected manner. And she had had 99.1° when she got up that morning—what was she likely to have by afternoon? The dressmaker confessed to the same temperature, but she on the contrary felt excited, tense, and restless, as though some important event were about to happen, which was certainly not the case; the excitation was purely physical, quite without emotional grounds.

---

[2] The Swedish Academy did not embrace the book wholeheartedly and it was stated that it was his debut novel *The Buddenbrooks* that Mann was praised for.

Yes, it is fiction and not reality. Although literature reflects humans and their culture, it is filtered through the mind of one writer, which is then the object of study rather than society itself. And while literature may reflect reality, we do not know if it is a representative reflection or not. Thomas Mann himself suffered from hypochondriasis, claiming that "all interest in illness and death is just another expression of interest in life."

Treatment with fresh air may or may not have been effective before the advent of antibiotics, but it is difficult to imagine a culture that more effectively causes a person to focus on their body, soul, and symptoms. I am deeply fascinated by sanatorium life and feel drawn to those alpine balconies and elegant lounges—while I don't necessarily think it would be good for me, it still feels enticing with rest cures, fresh air, conversation, drinks, reflection, and sublime, self-centered pondering in a mountain environment. Maybe a stay could stimulate new thoughts, somewhat as the sanatorium life seems to have contributed to Finnish author Edith Södergran's literary creativity? She spent a long time at Nummela's sanatorium in Uusimaa outside Helsinki but moved to Davos in 1912. She thought that life in Nummela was worse than in Davos where the cultural events were more numerous and social opportunities greater. Södergran wrote poems, enjoyed theatre and art exhibitions, attended concerts, and began studying Italian and English. She even fell in love with her doctor. I used to think of these things in the mornings while biking to work and looking up at Karolinska University Hospital's thoracic clinic with its white plastered terraces, before the buildings were demolished a few years ago. I would also definitely have preferred Davos (whose sanatoriums are now popular conference venues—my wife annoyingly often goes there, but the organizers seem to largely neglect the rest cures, deep psychology, and air baths) to Karolinska, considering both the view and the air pollution a few meters from the heavily trafficked road separating the hospital from Karolinska Institutet. I note while writing this, without thinking about it, that I have settled into an old wicker sofa on the sun deck of our cottage under a soft blanket. I suppose it will have to do.

So what do I mean by health in the distorted mirror of society? I am not referring to the peculiar qualities of sanatorium culture, but to the fact that we see, experience, and create our health experiences in the mirror that society holds up. The context in which we find ourselves offers a reflective surface and a framework within which we shape our perceived health. And it is a "fun house" mirror because the image can be distorted and contribute to an illusion about the body and its condition.

The view of sanatorium rest cures also reflects a past uncritical view of rest, far from today's debate about how inactivity can contribute to pain and overweight, and the fact that physical activity has anti-inflammatory properties. It is far from the insight that sick leave represents a risk in itself, although it may of course be a necessity. The sanatorium culture also reflects the view of health as a normal condition (despite Dr Krokowski's attitude that everyone is sick, if only given the time to look properly), which could be recaptured. We now know that inactivity is a factor in ill health, and we believe that too much focus on one's own body gives the brain's constructive working methods the opportunity to experience appropriate symptoms. We know that health is sensitive to context through learning and other placebo or nocebo mechanisms, through the brain's interpretation of the body, and through the behaviors with which we respond to this interpretation. It is not as simple as someone imagining that they are sick because it suggests that individuals would have great power to consciously invent ill health. It is more reasonable that some individuals unluckily fall victim to society's view of ill health in a process that, all things considered, is quite normal and happening in us all. The machinery is available in our brains. Hans Castorp symbolizes a person for whom society's view of health creates ill health.

Our contextual lives

Society and culture create an interpretive framework for our health experiences. Within this framework our flexible system of physical states can interpret, evaluate, and directly affect the condition. Do the symptoms correspond to a known diagnosis? Do the symptoms differ from what I expected given my age and what I demand from life? Am I really free from pain? Shouldn't one be tired if one has slept as little as I have? Are the symptoms compatible with work or social activities? Do I think resting would help me get healthy or would it be better to stay active? Are activities draining or energizing? Are there other more important behavioral goals that are competing with the motivation to rest and withdraw? As you read in Chapter 2, we start to build simple models for how the brain performs calculations in order to solve problems in which signal strength, motivation, learning, behavioral goals, reward, and expectation are central concepts. In Chapter 4 you read about signals that the body can send to the brain to pull an emergency brake and slow us down; and in Chapter 5, how calculations about infection risk can affect our attitudes toward other people through risk estimations based on assumptions, prejudices, and learning. In Chapters 6, 7, and 8, I described determinants of perceived health and the role society plays in conveying context and the culture's view of health in a way that affects our perception of our bodies and possible symptoms.

There is no doubt that the models will be rebuilt and refined for years to come. But if we look around the world and back at history, might we make observations that are consistent with these models and the functional flexibility through which our health seems to be computed? Let's start with a historical perspective.

The late Karin Johannisson, a past professor of the history of science and ideas, describes in a series of books and papers, diseases from a historic perspective. In particular, she highlights diffuse health conditions—states that seem to share a common "symptom pool." Depressed mood is one such symptom whose explanation and experience have occurred in many forms, and sometimes quite strange ones. In the 1600s, *lycanthropy* emerged as a kind of melancholy in which the sufferer experienced being, or being transformed into, a wolf.

A prime example of diffuse symptoms is fatigue. This symptom has also been described, explained, and experienced in a wide variety of ways at different times. Johannisson describes how fatigue has been explained in various ways throughout history, and a central notion of hers is that the description of the condition influences how the condition itself is shaped and experienced. The notion of fatigue caused by overexertion was an essential part of cultural analysis at the turn of the last century, where fatigue played the role of "the ever-present revenge goddess" of progress. After exertion, fatigue was eventually labelled *neurasthenia*, as the explanation was now based on nerves. The term stood for a physical weakness of the nerves. My grandfather Harald Berg, a perpetual student at Uppsala University, received a pleading letter in the spring of 1914 from a friend: a poet, songwriter, and artist called Olof Thunman. Thunman concluded the letter from his sickbed: "Send me a few lines immediately! It is absolutely necessary. I think I have nerves." I'm sure he really did have nerves, but I have a more prosaic view of this and apparently a more complex view of fatigue than the good Mr Thunman. But "having nerves" is a beautiful expression. Later in the twentieth century, chronic fatigue replaced neurasthenia, followed by burnout, and later exhaustion. Burnout seemed to initially affect women in subordinate positions, often in healthcare, but has spread to the IT industry and beyond and is seen as a sign of being dutiful and working too hard.

Suffering is considerable and diseases are real, despite the fact that diseases are not a neutral consequence of biological factors. Had the disease been a neutral consequence of a disease process (pathophysiology), we could have retained the biomedical model in which disease processes are what directly and exclusively explain suffering and disability.

Karin Johannisson demonstrates, through many examples, how society's values and social codes are reflected in diagnoses. Culturally conditioned ill health appears to arise in the intersection between medicine, society, and the individual, and derives its characteristics from a common group of diffuse symptoms such as fatigue, depression, and pain—symptoms that are also central to the sickness response. I would add that culturally conditioned ill health can hardly be a delimited entity, that is to say *only* conditioned by our context, and I therefore think that the often-used term "cultural diseases" is misleading. In addition, the influence of culture and society is obviously also part of more traditional diseases in which there are clear and known underlying disease processes. The contribution from culture is thus a part of the disease but does not normally define or explain it in its entirety. It likely plays a greater role in subjectively diffuse disease states in the same way that the placebo phenomenon may be present in all states of health and ill health, but has greater leeway in subjectively characterized states.

Instead of looking back in time, let's now look around the world and study cultural differences in how health is expressed and experienced. For many years, the medical anthropologist Lisbeth Sachs has made this her area of study. She emphasizes that it is "good to think with" other cultures. Through them we can spot our own way of looking at health and discover how our points of view are much less obvious than one might think.

Lisbeth Sachs' anthropological studies show, through concrete examples, how different cultures offer us diverse interpretive frameworks and thus context-bound experiences of one's own and others' health. We interpret information about disease processes based on our life experiences, and also based on a template that is naturally influenced by the culture, or the context, in which we live. Here, too, we see how it seems to affect the experience. Lisbeth Sachs lived close to Turkish women from Kulu in Anatolia and followed them when they migrated to Sweden. It seemed that their health experiences were changing in the new context, with new explanations and linguistic expressions. The women began to experience symptoms they had not previously had. They often viewed their health condition as deteriorating after coming to Sweden, and talked about "the Swedish pain" as a phenomenon they associated with life in Sweden.

One significant change for the Turkish immigrant women was that their newborn children survived to a greater extent than in the villages of Anatolia where child mortality was 25 percent in some areas, and several of the women reported that they gave birth to eight children, but that only five or six of them survived. In Sweden, more of their newborns survived, even though they had injuries at birth. There was a feeling that children born in Sweden were of "poorer quality," as one of the women put it. The women had difficulty taking care of disabled children, and in some cases didn't want to. Such children were God's children. The example seems to show how even the view of our own children's health is affected by cultural contexts.

It was not only factors that could be controlled or avoided, such as material conditions, that determined women's health, but also the social and cultural contexts. I imagine that, in many cases, the latter can be seen as positive determinants of health, but when they are not fulfilled—like after emigration—they lose their protective function. One's cultural perception of what health and illness are becomes important because people act in part based on their ideas, and health behaviors are a strong determinant of future health.

We can imagine how the perception of health affects behavior, such as when seeking care, taking prescriptions, and following healthy sleep and exercise habits; this even applies to the systems in the brain that protect against pain, draw attention to the body, or amplify symptoms. Lisbeth Sachs describes how, while living their traditional lives in Anatolia, the Turkish women are stoic, working at heavy chores well into pregnancy in spite of obvious infections and other challenges. However, in the new country, they seem to allow themselves to be more responsive to their symptoms and clearly suffer from head, stomach, or back pain. They say they have not had such symptoms in Kulu. Their approach to listening and attending to symptoms is influenced by the fact that they want to stay at home. In Sweden, they are given the opportunity to go on sick leave, and "that sickness fund" means that they can live a more traditional life in their small circle and avoid strangers, not least foreign men, outside the home. Rehabilitation is not a strong interest.

Not infrequently, the women travel back to their homeland to visit healers when they think their suffering is not understood in Sweden. After such trips, they often return to life in the suburb Tensta in better health. Lisbeth Sachs points out how knowledge about placebo makes it increasingly difficult to dismiss depictions of healing rituals and magic as mere anecdotes. Around the world, ways to help people feel better and be healthy vary, but common factors are how bodily healing processes are activated through trust and how rituals are created to maximize these effects.

Some of what we see illustrates bottom-up and top-down processes that are active even in terms of individual and specific disease states. In both historical and cultural variations in manifestations of ill health, we see a balance between these processes and some leeway in the brain's influence. The brain's top-down mechanisms are used to express society's values and explanatory models for each individual. One level concerns the pure interpretation of the signals from the rest of the body. This may have to do with how the signals are experienced and noticed, whether they lead to behavioral changes, and the symptoms you remember, describe to a healthcare provider, or report in a health questionnaire. Another level concerns how perceptions of health and illness, and what is useful or dangerous, affect not only the interpretation of symptoms but also the direct underlying physiological processes that form the basis of disease. We currently have some understanding of how placebo and nocebo work. This understanding is sufficient to conclude that the influence is real and undoubtably takes place. We discussed conditioning, placebo, and nocebo in Chapter 2, and mindset in Chapter 8. All of these processes are parts of the comprehensive machinery available to us to regulate health processes "from above." When discussing these phenomena, one can often hear that "experience can shape biology" or that "consciousness can affect the brain." But these expressions are nonsense and remnants of a dualistic model in which thoughts, feelings, and behaviors are believed to be distinct from the body. Can experience or thoughts shape biology? Of course, since they are biological processes in themselves. How else could it be, and why do we express ourselves as though psychological or perceived aspects are taking place in a parallel universe and not in our bodies?

When it comes to traditional emotional expressions, we understand from history and from current practices that societal and cultural norms are significant determinants. We know that normally reserved Swedes at times have reunited with old friends by throwing their arms around their necks, tears running down their faces while proclaiming their love. Or that the similarly restrained citizens let themselves go in church, speak in tongues, and tearfully profess their love for Jesus. We know that during periods it was considered good to cry with excitement, that this testified to one's sensitivity, and that being easily moved was a positive personal trait. During some periods it has been common for men to cry out of emotion, and during others, not. The expression has been turned on and off. In today's society, crying seems to decline more sharply after adolescence for men than for women.

We see great variation in how emotions are expressed, and how they are guided by context. It is likely that this also applies to physical symptoms even in a sickness response.[3] One can probably let oneself go in the sickness response and amplify it in a similar way as we can with happiness or grief. There is no fundamental difference between underlying traditional emotions (such as fear or joy) and the sickness response that makes this impossible. The challenge on an individual level is finding the balance between listening inward and paying attention outward. Both extremes can contribute to ill health.

In the 1970s, the American psychiatrist and anthropologist Robert Levy described a strange mix of sadness and illness in Tahitians. Levy claimed that the Tahitians lacked words to describe grief and that after losses, they did not describe themselves as sad, but instead as sick. According to Levy, grief was "hypocognized" and there were no doctrines and systems to categorize the emotion. In addition, expressing grief and sadness was inappropriate in many contexts as it was considered good for a dying person

---

[3] A person I met who was active as a medium was interested in just the same things as I am regarding bodily expressions and their variation, but our explanations were dissimilar. She reported that if she had a cold, and let herself be taken over by a spirit she had a very close relation with, the symptoms of the cold disappeared.

to laugh. Grief after death could prevent the soul from leaving the body. Together with the lack of vocabulary and thought structures around grief, the only alternative was to "somatize" it—that is, to alter the reaction so that it was experienced in the body. The condition was experienced as illness or fatigue. The empiricist in me—which I would call my true self if I still thought there was one, but social psychology has hit me hard—recalls that these kinds of historical and cultural examples are merely anecdotal in nature. They seem to corroborate the occurrence of top-down phenomena in health processes but are not subject to experimental control. The examples here may have been caused by something completely different, but the "pattern collector" in me found and highlighted them as evidence of a particular model of thought.

From the controlled experiments we can perform, we can make predictions about historical and cultural variations. If these assumptions are true, variations should be similar to the ones I have described in these examples.

Rapidly changing ill health

The conditions that make people sick and die have changed significantly over the last century. Because the disease panorama is different, the requirements for preventive measures and ways of measuring health, functional level, and efficiency in healthcare need to be adapted. This is a major challenge, and major changes are needed. We are seeing a rapid shift in perspective: from contagious infectious diseases to non-communicable diseases (NCDs). These include a large group of diseases, but those that contribute most to premature death are cardiovascular disease, cancer, diabetes, and chronic lung disease. One of the chronic lung diseases is asthma, which can be allergic in nature, along with several other allergic conditions. Allergies are the most common NCDs in most regions of the world, and those that debut first in life. Around 30 percent of the world's population is estimated to suffer from allergies, so if we add "newer" conditions—such as autism, attention disorders, lupus, bowel disease, multiple sclerosis, or obesity—it is no longer a matter of whether you or your family members and friends suffer from these, but which of these conditions are present in your immediate circle. A one-sided, old-fashioned biomedical model fits this new disease panorama even worse than it fit the one we had before.

Global disease burden (measured as "years lived with disability") is dominated by non-communicable rather than infectious diseases. For the past three decades, back pain, depression, and headache disorders have prevailed as some of the leading causes of years lived with disability. Other pain problems, diabetes, and anxiety disorders are other important contributors to this not very honorable list. The figures for years lived with disability have decreased more slowly than the death toll over time—it thus contributes to an older population living with chronic diseases. In addition, individuals often suffer from more than one condition. Health and medical services therefore face a real challenge adjusting to caring for a population that lives longer but has more disabilities and multiple illnesses.

The fact that infection is now a less severe cause of ill health than before could mean that the mechanisms I describe in this book, with inflammation at the center, are no longer relevant. However, this is not the case—quite the opposite. Chronic low-grade inflammation is involved in almost all NCDs and is a common denominator in the main causes of disability and premature death. It shows, among other things, how clearly integrated the inflammatory system is with other physiological systems, including the nervous system, and that it is not just part of a defense against external infectious agents. Since it responds to danger, both protecting against dangers and inherently posing a threat in itself, it is central to homeostatic processes (which have to do with maintaining balance) in the body. So in terms of chronic diseases, it comes as no surprise that inflammation is involved both as a defense and cause of NCDs and contributes to functional impairment. And while we should not try to explain everything with inflammation, we do see a strong common denominator in the classic symptoms of NCDs, including pain, fatigue, and depression.

It is suspected, in several health conditions, that the inflammatory system does not appropriately shut down after activation. I have emphasized that it is an important survival system during emergencies, but that there are also risks involved, especially if the system is not downregulated when the task is hopefully resolved. Chronic low-grade inflammation is thought to have a connection to negative behavioral symptoms in many conditions.

In addition to inflammation, there is another important common denominator among NCDs in that they are lifestyle-related. In fact, they are linked by four common risk factors: tobacco, alcohol, unhealthy eating habits, and insufficient physical activity. This means that there is a huge opportunity within healthcare to transition to more effective prevention-oriented care that prevents ill health and thus both suffering and sick leave. But the challenge is great—not least in poorer countries, which are not spared from the strong increase in NCDs. And in the same way, it is a challenge in richer countries, not only to change the healthcare system, but also to ensure that the distribution of health and illness does not become even more unequally distributed among social groups. Subjective perceived social status, like both objective social status and self-rated health, is a good predictor of future ill health.

Today's and yesterday's health systems, with their biomedical orientation, fit poorly with today's disease panorama because people must live a long time with chronic illnesses, while they want and need to live as they did before. In addition, since ill health is so strongly linked to lifestyle, healthcare must to a greater extent be preventive in nature and be better at achieving behavioral objectives. Factors such as lifestyle, behavioral changes, coping strategies, psychological treatments, and subjective health measures are becoming increasingly important in the new disease landscape.

The new hidden diseases—you could be one of the victims!

At least, if you believe the headlines. They are effective at selling single copies based on our concerns about illness. It is easy to become fixated on health issues and to obey the urge to direct a spotlight on our own bodies, or even the brain for that matter. The health alarms are endless. We know that excessive attention to physical symptoms poses a risk to health and well-being, but can trying to live too healthy a life be a risk factor in itself? The term orthorexia (which is not a diagnosis) has been coined to denote an individual who is excessively fixated on a healthy lifestyle.

If demands are high or unrealistic, it is easy to feel unsuccessful and anxious. An orthorectic individual compulsively follows a diet that is often restrictive and lacks scientific support. It is difficult to follow very strict dietary requirements, and failure to do so leads to concerns about illness, anxiety, and shame. Therefore as a concept, it is related to health anxiety. The term orthorexia is close to the area of eating disorders, and is less associated with excessive fixation on other health behaviors like sleep and physical activity.

The many scientifically ill-founded methods of treating or preventing illness often do quite well commercially, despite their inferior evidence base. Much of the health industry is controlled by the free market and not based on secure ways of developing knowledge, which is troubling in itself. In the preface to a book, Edzard Ernst, a professor of complementary medicine, and his colleagues asked themselves what impact scientific support for a particular method had on popular health literature. They pulled down from their shelves seven books on complementary and alternative medicine to see if methods were recommended based on available evidence. In these particular books (there was no representative selection, they were picked haphazardly), complementary methods with scientific support were *not* recommended. On the other hand, many other methods were recommended, even for serious conditions, and here they seemed to be selected at random. For HIV/AIDS there were 69 different recommended treatments, and 89 for diabetes! But there were many more extreme examples, and the list was topped by cancer (133), arthritis (131), and addiction (120 different treatments). In a compilation of 685 connections between different treatments and conditions, only seven were estimated to be based on good evidence. Although established healthcare should always be based on the best available scientific evidence (something that, in reality, is far from true) and many patients expect this, it is clear that a whole stand-alone market can successfully manage without caring about scientific support. This is unfortunate because the scientific method is better than other methods for producing sustainable knowledge.

The way society values health likely influences what the various degrees of self-rated health mean. Although we envisage a continuous scale between very good and very poor health, it is likely that individuals assign different qualities, not just degrees of difference, to good and poor health. Good health can be seen by many as a normal condition or a baseline. Remaining on such a baseline needs no explanation, while departing from the baseline must have a specific cause and require an explanation, as the philosopher Georg Henrik von Wright and others have argued. The definition of "baseline" thus influences the perception of one's health through the assessment of how good one's health is in relation to what one might expect.

Capturing patients' health

Because subjective health factors are so important from the perspective of suffering and the connection to future illness, there are good reasons to ask questions directly to patients and to systematically collect information. A large movement around patient-reported outcome measures (PROMs) has swept the globe. In these measures, health status reports come directly from patients without the measures being interpreted by healthcare providers. In studies, measures have also been developed to gauge how healthcare works by creating overall measures based on

PROMs. This is needed because efficiency and care content can vary greatly across providers and regions. If the care is inefficient at one healthcare provider or in one region, that is a good reason for patients to stay away. And when healthcare organizations see that their results are worse than others, there are strong reasons to review their routines. The trend toward increased measurement of the value of patient care, both in terms of cure and other outcome measures, drives changes in healthcare and patient satisfaction. There are many reasons for systematic and coordinated measurement of the value of patient care, and some are quite concrete. In addition to increased treatment compliance, improved symptom control and better life quality are associated with reduced costs and use of healthcare resources. Furthermore, healthcare based on patient value spurs momentum to reorient care toward health maintenance and improvement rather than merely reacting to illness after the fact. WHO emphasizes that the transition to a person-centered healthcare system with continuous measurement of patient value is important to obtain cost-effective and sustainable healthcare, which, despite great successes, is difficult to claim we have today. With the new-age spectrum of ill health, the transition to healthcare that contains PROMs as well as modernized preventive care becomes more important. I am also reminded here of research findings on how self-reported outcome measures can be stronger predictors of mortality than those obtained through laboratory tests or physical examinations.

When important care data is collected in a structured and automated way, it represents what is called a quality register. This data can be used to evaluate the effectiveness of healthcare and identify regions or hospitals where healthcare results are better or below average. There are many examples of how such registers have been used successfully to improve care and survival in various types of disease including cancer, orthopedics, and diabetes.

As we shall see, a further benefit of registering quality measures and making them available is of a more democratic nature and applies to the right to information about care content and outcomes.

Treatment of mental illness

If it is easy to point out weaknesses in somatic care, then it is even easier to see deficiencies in the treatment of mental illness. This cannot be justified by supposing that the proportion of people in need of mental healthcare is a smaller and perhaps less significant part of the total number in need of care. According to the WHO, depression is one of the leading contributing causes of disease burden in the world. In primary care, it is usually said that about one-third have problems that are primarily of a psychosocial nature, but many other diseases also include behavioral aspects because they are related to lifestyle. In addition, people with mental illness are major consumers of somatic care, with an excessive mortality of about 50 percent compared to people with correspondingly severe conditions but without mental illness.

So then we fire off a set of appropriate cures, including lifestyle modification and psychological treatment, in addition to pharmacologically oriented psychiatric treatment where justified, right? And prevention where possible in order to save money and suffering by preventing ill health from occurring? Hardly. Undertreatment is enormous. In the United States and within the EU, less than one-third of those affected by mental illness receive healthcare, and those figures are far worse than those for common physical diseases. The brain, that is affected in mental illness, is of course a part of the body as well, but in some ways the suffering that belongs to our mental life is measured with another yardstick. The undertreatment of mental illness could be explained to a certain extent if there were no good treatments, but that is not the case. For the most common conditions there is psychological treatment, backed by strong scientific evidence, that is therefore recommended as the first choice of care in many countries. We know that the availability of this effective care is generally low. But in many cases, we have too little control over what treatments patients receive for which diagnoses, from which therapists with which education, whether full treatments are given or whether they are minimized to reduce costs, exactly how much patients improve, and whether the improvements last. After all, we have many indications of poor accessibility and implementation. It is possible to improve all of these things through relatively simple means. The knowledge is there, ready to be utilized, but major organizational changes are needed.

In fact, such changes have been made in a very large British project called IAPT (Improving Access to Psychological Therapies). The principle behind the program is to implement guidelines for the treatment of depression and anxiety—the most common types of mental illness. In order to properly implement the guidelines, therapists were trained in specific treatments. By "properly" I mean that treatments should be performed in the same way and by people with the same education as in the scientific trials on which the guidelines were based. This means, for example, that the entire treatment involves a certain number of sessions, let's say 10, for a certain condition, and no fewer. To give half the treatment then, as they say in the IAPT program, is analogous to telling the patient, "You are entitled to one hour of heart surgery."

The starting point for the British government's investment in evidence-based mental healthcare was a health economics analysis conducted by psychologist David Clark and economist Richard Layard. They argued that healthcare savings would exceed costs for properly performed treatment, as would savings for the government treasury. Half of the patients were estimated to have recovered after treatment, that is, to have been successfully treated, in addition to the majority who improved, even if they were not considered to be fully recovered. The claim that it is too expensive to use psychological treatment is therefore not true. On the contrary, it is extremely expensive not to do so. We simply can't afford not to. After presenting these calculations, the British government invested hundreds of millions of pounds to reduce suffering and save money. The program was rolled out and made available in most of the country. Almost half of the patients became healthy and many more improved.

The IAPT program is based on implementing guidelines, which may be easier said than done. The guidelines are based on the evaluation of studies in order to determine the level of support for a certain treatment or condition. If the support is strong, it is reflected in treatment guidelines—that is, in comprehensive instructions on how a condition should be treated. However, the transition from guidelines to care can be problematic when implementation takes place in an environment of unclear governance, insufficient knowledge and resources, and with ideologically colored views on preferred treatments that are not based on scientific evidence. In the British example, therapists were trained and units approved to ensure that the treatments were performed properly. Throughout the program, an important principle was followed to make it easier to evaluate how well the guidelines were implemented and how effective the care was. Each unit working with the program gathered data on characteristics of the treated patients (such as diagnosis, age, and gender), the patients' own evaluations, and outcome measures relating to treatment effectiveness. Anyone could then see how a particular region or individual care unit was performing. This kind of data transparency has many advantages. One is purely democratic: sharing information with other citizens, regardless of position or class, and making it easily accessible. Gathering PROMs contributed to the transfer of power to the users. Perhaps this is especially important in an area such as mental health, where afflicted individuals can hardly be expected to navigate through effective care systems in a timely manner.

Patients' voices can be heard if data is made available, and prospective patients can choose care based on more information. In addition to this democratic advantage, there is also an opportunity to improve the quality of care when data is made available. Through IAPT, it was discovered that the variation in efficiency was too great among different units. While some units performed fantastically well, there were others that were far below the expected 50 percent recovery rate (that is, the number of patients who do not meet the criteria for a post-treatment diagnosis). To understand what happened at the low-performing units, data and care were analyzed. The common denominator turned out to be that they did not strictly adhere to treatment processes, but instead went "off piste." These results are interesting in that they indicate the importance of adhering to treatment protocols.

Although the importance of clinical experience and skill should not be underestimated, there are many reasons to believe that exaggerated confidence in one's own ability to tailor treatments reduces effectiveness. Not surprisingly, a well-documented cognitive source of error called "overconfidence" is in play here. The phenomenon is particularly common in political, religious, and ideological views, and an ideological bias regarding views on psychological treatment is evident. Making decisions is difficult, and we often have unreasonably strong feelings and beliefs about our ability to absorb large amounts of information and use it to make objective judgments. When making such assessments and when uncertainty is great, our strong feeling should be taken with a grain of salt. This is the case when treating mental illness. When I see how healthcare policy is conducted in this area, I get somewhat frustrated. Act on the data and the overall evidence, I want to say—they exist and they speak through our patients and for their best interest.

Consequently, with regard to the less well-performing IAPT units, the guidelines were more poorly implemented than in the better-functioning units. When this was discovered, changes could be initiated, after which the units came up to par. At present, 51 percent of the patients have recovered following treatment, and two-thirds have shown consistent improvement.

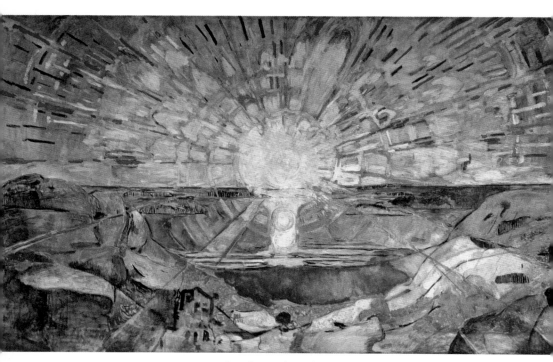

Edvard Munch's "The sun"

© O. Vaering/Bridgeman Images

10

PERHAPS IT'S NOT THAT BAD?

I f you're reading this book, you are presumably a curious person who is driven by an interest in how things are connected. You have read about strange new brain research where big leaps are taken in our understanding of how experience is related to activity in our brains. You have also read about the rapid increase in knowledge of how we defend ourselves against illness, and how behavior and experience are important to increase the level of protection and to adapt to environmental demands. How can we use this knowledge to feel better, and is there a risk that too much or incorrect knowledge will hurt us? How quickly does knowledge increase, and how long will it take until we have a reasonable understanding of the brain's functions?

It is somewhat similar to looking up at a high mountain from a lift. You can see that the mountain is mighty and that it is far to the summit, but you rapidly get closer, knowing you will soon be there. Translating this to research about humans' inner lives, will we understand the brain's biology in a way that matches psychology's knowledge about behavior in perhaps a decade or two? Hardly. As everyone who has ascended a mountain has noticed, a new and even mightier summit will likely become visible beyond the one you initially saw. It may continue on like that as you begin to realize that your starting view obscured the full picture, and that the powerful mountain was only the first in a series of mountains—or perhaps in a full mountain chain. This is also a probable scenario when it comes to understanding how our brain works. The phenomenon of overestimating your degree of knowledge, and believing that you have access to all relevant information, is well known in psychology. What you see is all there

The Inflamed Feeling. Mats Lekander, Oxford University Press. © Mats Lekander 2022.
DOI: 10.1093/oso/9780198863441.003.0010

is, as Daniel Kahneman has expressed it. Machinery is always there to help you jump to conclusions. And even if progress is considerable, we are very far from having reasonable knowledge about how the brain works. If—and let's be clear—*if* the brain is a system that can understand itself at all. Perhaps a much more advanced brain would be needed to understand our current one. The tools we currently have at our disposal are amazing and give rise to dizzying experiences—like seeing another human's brain work—but they are still very blunt.

I previously felt relatively alone among psychoneuroimmunology researchers who were well versed on the latest developments in cognitive neuroscience. Luckily, those days are long gone. Neuroimaging has almost become the meat and potatoes of human studies of connections between the immune system and behavior. Integration is the key word here, especially because psychoneuroimmunology, as we hoped, has become part of the common biological, and often psychological, discourse. Perspectives on inflammation and its influence on brain function, pain signalling, or behavior in general, are soon to be included in nearly any scientific meeting touching upon basic physiology, psychology, or related psychiatric or pain research. It is remarkable that just a few decades ago, the dominant scientific view of the immune system was of a self-regulating system of little relevance to the brain. The pendulum has now swung back, and "everybody" seems to be interested in inflammation. Understanding these neuroinflammatory processes will hardly shed light on all health-related problems, but it is clearly relevant because, as a part of the generalized sickness response, it is involved in many different conditions.

Perhaps you are the kind of person who reads about health because you are looking for ways to improve your own health. Your health is good, your doctor says, but that's not your experience. Or maybe your doctor's views coincide with your own regarding either physical or psychological concerns. If so, I have no reason to say that it's not that bad, per the title of this chapter. But I will say so anyway for two reasons. The first is that, in many social classes in many cultures, health is getting better and better. Those of us (and I view myself as belonging to this group) who have good or reasonably good health are common. The second reason is that, for many people, *worrying* about health is a very big part of the problem. This can relate to worrying about being or becoming sick, fear of pain or of moving because it will hurt, or fear of the danger of sleep problems (which in a vicious circle leads to more sleep problems). The worry could also relate to concern that the bodily signals one experiences in connection to fatigue, stress, or simply being a human being, are in fact symptoms of disease. Anxiety is a common burden that negatively influences our well-being, our functioning, and—by extension—our objective health.

I'd like to dwell on the group of people who view their health as poor but who cannot get it confirmed by a health professional. If this sounds like you, you may experience symptoms that your doctor cannot reasonably explain. And I feel fairly sure that your doctor has not been able to help you in a satisfying way. This may be due in part to medicine's restricted knowledge or diagnostic methods. What we know about health is not all there is, right? And subjective experiences should not be dismissed, as we have learned earlier in this book. One of the reasons is that the way we experience health is a good predictor of future objectively verifiable health, and this also holds true in large statistical calculations in which objectively verified health factors, such as diagnoses, are taken into account. The subjective experience provides information beyond that of a biomedical nature. The movement advocating for patient-reported health outcome measures is based not only on empathy, but on the viewpoint that suffering should be taken seriously and considered together with hard facts related to objective outcomes.

If the level of worry about your health is too strong, allow me to raise another question. We do not really know why subjective health ratings on a statistical level predict future objective health. Part of the explanation probably depends on the fact that poor health experiences are linked to behaviors that increase the risk of future ill health. If worry or anxiety are part of the problem—and that is clearly the case in many diagnoses—there are ways to treat it. Viewing one's health in a realistic perspective, and using active strategies to manage society's ill-health fixation, is not a bad approach.

Sometimes two dimensions of health are described. One dimension is the biomedical one connected to diagnoses, and the other is the subjective health experience—in other words, the presence or absence of disease in one dimension and one's personal experience of health in the other. With increased interdisciplinary knowledge, the subjective perspective has emerged as an important aspect that the healthcare sector must consider to be effective. One negative consequence of health fixation and worry, which pushes people to look inward in search of symptoms, is that we risk pushing people downward in the subjective dimension, and thereby potentially into becoming "ill" in the disease dimension. It is possible, but not proven, that this applies to somatic diseases. However, it seems to apply to mental illness in which these kinds of processes amplify worry and anxiety and contribute to the development of a disabling disorder.

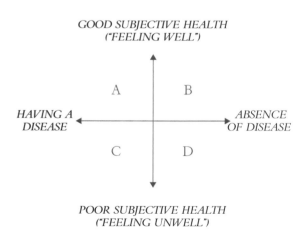

FIGURE 10.1 Illustration of the two dimensions of health: The biomedical one related to diagnosis, and the subjective health experience.

The mechanisms of discontent

I have pointed out how many health measures have moved in a positive direction for many of the world's population groups. I am not unaware of the instability causing hardships in parts of the world, of superstitious outlooks on life and irrational beliefs that spread, or of drug abuse, violence, inequities, and insecurity which can occur even among those who are financially stable. Likewise, I am not unaware of the considerable problems of mental illness, how it is treated, and perhaps more to the point, how it is not treated.

Still, there are reasons to be optimistic, or at least to allow oneself to see improvements that have taken place—this is also probably so where you live, if I base my assumptions on typical readers of popular science books. Can we see these improvements? Would seeing them be of any benefit? I believe so.

Some might say that it's not the cards you're dealt, but how you play them that counts. There is a grain of truth to this expression. I have highlighted the importance of top-down processes and coping strategies in this book, and I have also explained several mechanisms behind these processes. One's approach to ill health, when it appears, has some irrefutable impact on well-being and function.

A variation of this expression could be that it's not the cards you're dealt, *or* how you play them, but the cards that *others* are dealt that counts. If we believe we have reason to think that we should be unhappy with our situation, we are pushed toward change, which is completely logical from an evolutionary perspective. The reason for the feeling of discontent may be a change in a certain direction, rather than our absolute level of health or living conditions. In this way, it is the direction that is critical—a deterioration gives rise to negative emotions (which motivate behavioral change), and improvement gives rise to positive emotions (which do not motivate behavior change). The emotion is a driving force. It is reasonable that this phenomenon also applies to health. Dopamine neurons in the midbrain are involved in reward so that they can govern behavior through learning. Most of these neurons are in fact activated if the reward is *larger* than expected, but respond with *reduced* activity if the reward is smaller than expected. Furthermore, some neurons in the frontal lobe respond primarily to the difference between obtained and expected reward. If health changes in the right direction, and more than we expected, this translates to a reward value that is not necessarily related to *where* on a scale between poor and good health we are situated.

An effective way to know whether we should be content or not is to compare oneself with others—is my situation or my health better or worse than it should be when I compare myself to my fellow human beings? We know that both humans and (other) animals can be very sensitive, so the reward value of something (say salary) can change quickly if we discover that other people are getting larger rewards (like a higher salary for the same work). Translated to health, it would mean poor perceived health in relation to how I, according to myself, *should* be. There are good reasons to believe that self-ratings like this are actually performed in an active, dynamic, and comparative way. And translated to neuro-lingo, believing that I ought to be in just as good shape as someone else I am comparing myself to is related to a lack of signal from the frontal lobes saying that everything is good enough and that nothing should be changed—an "everything is ok signal." The absence of such signals is believed to motivate behavior and to release a "break" on how easily the cortex can be stimulated to act.

Throughout this book I have given examples of how the brain's handling of bodily signals can be compared to how it manages signals received from the surrounding world, and how in this way we can better understand health. If you remember Figure 1.5 from Chapter 1, depicting the Ebbinghaus illusion, the inner circle appears smaller if it is surrounded by larger rather than smaller circles. Imagine your health as an inner circle of a certain size. It will appear to be better or worse depending on the context and the size of the surrounding circles. It is hard to free yourself from the power of the illusion even when you know how it works. Context impacts the interpretation of one's own body in a way that we have only just begun to explore in the scientific world.

Feelings of the kind that make us act when something is wrong are needed for survival and for making beneficial decisions. We know that the inability to involve feelings and emotional signals in our decisions can lead to personal problems, something which can be observed as an effect of certain lesions in the frontal lobes. We are without a doubt in deep trouble without our emotions, but emotional states and the force with which they are expressed do not tell us much about how the world is constructed. So the strength of my convictions should be taken with a grain of salt in relation to how well I believe it represents the truth. Signals sent to the brain are diffuse and must be interpreted; they often guide our behavior in a general sense (that is, encouraging us to approach, avoid, change strategy, or continue) rather than explaining or "depicting." Sometimes I contemplate how I appraise my own health and degree of well-being. Can I "see" what is good, and how do I handle that which is less good? My subjective health is reasonably better than that of the beggar I may pass on the street, but how many generations would I need to go back in my own family tree to find individuals who generally[1] have worse health, objectively or subjectively, than that of the beggar whose suffering I have such trouble coping with? In such cases, I make an assumption about worse health in earlier

---

[1] I write "generally" because each person has a number of ancestors whose number grows exponentially for each past generation. It is difficult to know which ancestor you would choose if you did not think in terms of an average. My mind boggles when I think of it, but I have (at most) over a million ancestors in a straight ascending line 20 generations above me, which would amount to about 500 years back in time. "At most" is an important qualification since the same people occur several times when people who are related to one another have children. If this phenomenon did not occur, the number of ancestors a few dozen generations back in time would be higher than the number of people on the entire earth at a given time. But I still get the feeling that what I have become accustomed to seeing as "related" is a concept that makes no sense unless one is referring to the absolute near time, which from a geological time perspective is completely negligible. I am certainly a carrier of genes in a river of life (*River out of Eden*), as Richard Dawkins put it, but my clannishness (which is still only moderately strong) gets another blow not only from thinking in geological time, but also just thinking back to the Middle Ages. Yet my ancestors speak through me, as I previously pointed out, in that the genes I inherited from them make me *want* to do things that they *had* to do in order to survive and to make those genes function in my body so many years later.

generations based on knowledge about increased longevity, reduced infant mortality, contemporary healthcare, access to food, and improved general life conditions, with fewer people over time belonging to the group experiencing very poor health.

I don't want to underestimate other peoples' suffering in modern society. I do not claim that mental illness, addiction, violence, or social pressures are uncommon. All of these phenomena are sufficient to cause suffering even in a society with better financial security, more free time, and more automated assistance with laundry, transportation, and cooking. What good are such modern benefits if mom is an alcoholic who doesn't care for me?

Back to mindset

One concrete reason for believing that things are not necessarily as bad as one might think is the knowledge that one's attitude toward burdens like stress, lack of sleep or shift work, can make it all worse. One can thus have an exaggerated fear that is more related to what one thinks or has learned about the body than the danger itself, and which makes bad things seem worse. At a glance, this appears just as reassuring as the claim that the dog who sniffs you in the crotch will only bite if you are scared. However, since many misconceptions exist about the risks of stress and lack of sleep, some of the added risk from worry might be reduced through information. A further argument is that the fear and anxiety associated with a disorder are often part of the problem, so if you get help with that, which you can for chronic pain or tinnitus, the situation can prove less troublesome than you thought it was.

I have briefly mentioned that the effects of stress can be affected by whether one views stress as dangerous or helpful. In fact, there is a reasonably large amount of literature on this. Researchers have often used short instructions to try to affect the way people look at stress. Instead of seeing the physiological stress response as negative and harmful, the researcher emphasizes how it is helpful during challenging situations, and that it has evolved to help people in trying times. It is important to point out that such an instruction can be given without lying. The acute stress response undoubtedly has adaptive functions, although it can be perceived as unpleasant. These studies have been shown to result in improved school test scores or better performances during oral presentations. The studies are done in slightly different ways—as it should be—comparing positive instructions with negative ones, with no instructions at all, or with prompts to simply ignore feelings of stress. In some cases, an impact on biologically measured outcomes has been captured as well. In a way, these studies confirm something that has been known for a long time: that one's appraisal of the burden, and the resources one possesses, affect the stress response. But this knowledge gains greater power and depth these days.

One reason why this perspective is important is the easy access to and broad dissemination of information on how dangerous stress is. Unbalanced information about stress is frequently spread by the media, through lecturers, in popular science books, and on the internet, where positive short-term consequences are forgotten, and where the risks of long-term stress are often exaggerated. Another reason why the perspective of appraisal is relevant lies in how knowledge about emotional regulation has increased, not least regarding our understanding of how the brain modulates emotional responses. And this new knowledge is of course relevant for stress as well.

An active interpretation can also apply to symptoms such as worry and unpleasant thoughts, making such symptoms sensitive to manipulation. Shrewd researchers collected baseline data about peoples' symptoms, but then misinformed the subjects that they had rated some symptoms higher than they actually did. More than half of the participants did not detect that they were misinformed. When followed up a week later, blinded participants now rated the same symptoms as higher—that is, they reported stronger symptoms in the direction of the misinformation! Many similar studies have been performed regarding opinions or perception of the outer world, and obviously, the intensity of symptoms can vary according to our beliefs.

Other studies reinforce the impression that we are not very good at monitoring interoceptive information, that is, "messages" from the inner world. It is thus open to influence from society and cultures, in a way that will ultimately affect how we experience our bodies and our health. A negative impact of (mis)belief may also be observed on objective measures of health over time, as indicated by some epidemiological studies. And a smaller study, compared to the epidemiological studies, suggests that people who state that they think stress is dangerous to health later report slightly more physical symptoms six to eight weeks after the measurement.

In fact, your situation may be less dangerous than you think. If we think of public health as a continuum from poor to good health, where a certain proportion of the population has diagnosable symptoms, my hypothesis is that today's approach to health, stress, and sleep propel some fairly healthy people across the boundary to the group that fulfills diagnostic criteria. Not only from quadrant A to C or B to D in Figure 10.1 shown earlier in the chapter, but also from B to C.

A positive side of what I have illustrated in this section and in previous chapters is that it comes with clear healing potential,[2] as opposed to a belief in fixed boundaries between sick and healthy brains, bodies, and behaviors.

Changing one's behavior

For those of you who want to change your behavior, my advice is this: follow scientific evidence. Scientific literature is neither perfect nor complete, but there is no doubt that the scientific method takes us closer to the truth. In most cases, you will therefore receive the best help if you follow scientifically sound advice. It is natural to ask if you as an individual are perhaps an

---

[2] The regulatory perspective I am talking about is based on a *dimensional* perspective of health or emotional phenomena. It is founded in the fact that there is most often not a categorical difference between sick or healthy, but that a phenomenon such as anxiety exists in all people to varying degrees. The opposite view is called a discrete or categorical view.

exception. Is it possible that I, as an individual, would get better help from a method that has worse scientific support than one that has better support because it seems reasonable in some way? That cannot be excluded, but there is almost never any way to find out if you belong to the minority that is better served by a method with less support as compared to the majority that is better helped by a method with stronger support. And as we saw in the example of English mental healthcare, therapists overestimate their ability to "feel" which method is best for a particular individual, and this bias also applies to patients.

If you want to change behavior and get healthier, you should use sources that follow scientific methods and that are based on reviews and research compilations rather than individual research results (which may be wrong) or claims that just "feel" right. Products for self-care or treatments that do not match basic assumptions about how humans and nature work should be avoided because you are entitled to both a placebo *and* a "real" effect. Self-help books have, in some cases, good scientific support and may contain the same treatment you would get from going to an expensive therapist. However, the requirements needed for you to complete an entire treatment on your own are of course higher than if you have support and a social contract with a therapist. A health anxiety management lesson that can be applied more generally is that one's situation does not necessarily need to be as bad as one might think. Needless to say, this consideration applies once relevant health examinations have been done by traditional healthcare providers. But if worry and anxiety are part of the problem and are thought to be too great, there are techniques to reduce them.

Our bodies are not silent but give rise to sensations, and to what we sometimes want to call symptoms, even when we are completely healthy. This is what psychologist Gordon Asmundson calls "body noise," which entails unexpected and sometimes unwelcome signals from the body. If you sit down and focus on your body, it is natural that you will experience such noise. The experiences can relate to fatigue, perhaps shortness of breath, pain, tension, or even physical well-being. Such noise in the body, at least the kind we perceive as negative, increases at higher anxiety or stress levels or when changing routines. It may be related to inactivity or may occur together with minor (harmless) health conditions. The role that this body noise plays in your well-being, and how much attention you pay to the signals, all depend on numerous factors related to your definition of "dangerous" and "harmless" and to the environment. Anthropologist Lisbeth Sachs describes a number of phenomena about how we relate to our bodies, including how the state of flow is associated with the absence of body awareness, in that the body and its possible ailments are completely forgotten during the creative and focused state that characterizes flow. In flow, attention is thus selective, but instead of directing much attention toward the body, it is directed so strongly outward that the body "disappears."

One aspect that makes health concerns worse is repeatedly checking and paying close attention to bodily changes. The same applies to repeatedly checking one's health status with healthcare providers, or reading about health issues in the media and on the internet. Avoiding situations that make you worried about health reinforces concerns and therefore worry. It is exactly the same phenomenon as in many other health conditions—avoidant behaviors that one performs to reduce anxiety in the short run in fact sustain it over a longer period of time. As I mentioned in Chapter 8, exposure can be used to reduce a problem: if you are exposed to the discomfort gradually, and under safe conditions, the nervous system can learn that a behavior, situation, or place is not dangerous. When the health concerns are great, this can be quite helpful. One way is to confront bodily symptoms that make you anxious, and another is to expose yourself to situations that contribute to anxiety. Confronting bodily signals and symptoms is simply an interoceptive exposure. There are a number of techniques to get these internal signals started, for example by swallowing four times as quickly as you can, breathing through a straw for a while, or straining one's muscles hard for one minute. This kind of exposure overlaps with panic anxiety treatments in which patients may believe that their hearts will be injured if they continue beating at an increased rate. To prevent this, those who are affected try to do whatever it takes to avoid the things that elevate their anxiety and heart rates. Challenging this belief with a reality test, lead by a therapist, means that patients cannot escape from situations that cause discomfort, thereby increasing their pulse; they then discover that their hearts did not stop and that they survived the strong bodily signals. Similarly, situations that provoke fear and reinforce health anxiety can be challenged and combined with so called *response prevention* so that worry and anxiety decrease.

So why is it so difficult to change behavior? One reason lies in how the reward system works, specifically in conflicts between short-term and long-term benefits. Avoidance behavior, or eating a chocolate cake you had previously decided to save, provides an immediate reward. However, following a predetermined action plan provides delayed rewards in the distant future. Quick feedback is much more effective at influencing behaviors, so it is difficult for a long-term reward to win over its immediately available cousin. Maybe it is rewarding, even in the short term, to follow a new action plan when one has just begun to change a behavior (how good I was for exercising for so long!), but this value diminishes quickly. Behavioral change should therefore be organized, if possible, in ways that make it rewarding both in the short term and long term. The reward system is a tough enemy to fight. The funny thing is that, with a little perseverance, you eventually reach a point where the new behavior becomes seriously rewarding.

It feels good to have improved one's health, not least the health one consciously experiences in both the body and in one's head. And as we know, we can enjoy the direction of the change—the plain fact that it is getting better—no matter where we start on our own scale of perceived health.

You are populated by bacteria and parasites, by white blood cells that negotiate security threats with your brain. You hear your ancestors' voices telling you about life and death through your genes, and you are influenced by societal and personal values so that you can choose to ignore bodily signals or fully experience health challenges that absorb all your attention. Despite all this, it is still your inner life we are talking about.

You are the meeting place for these forces that govern your health.

REFERENCES

Preface

Flegr J, Lenochová P, Hodný Z, Vondrová M. Fatal attraction phenomenon in humans: Cat odour attractiveness increased for toxoplasma-infected men while decreased for infected women. *PLoS Negl Trop Dis*. 2011;5(11):e1389.

Manga-González MY, González-Lanza C, Cabanas E, Campo R. Contributions to and review of dicrocoeliosis, with special reference to the intermediate hosts of Dicrocoelium dendriticum. *Parasitology*. 2001;123(Suppl):S91–114.

Swain F. *How to make a zombie: The real life (and death) science of reanimation and mind control*. London: Oneworld Publications; 2013.

Zhang Y, Träskman-Bendz L, Janelidze S, et al. Toxoplasma gondii immunoglobulin G antibodies and nonfatal suicidal self-directed violence. *J Clin Psychiatry*. 2012;73(8):1069–76.

1. What does the brain know about the outside world?

Andersen BL, Winawer J. Image segmentation and lightness perception. *Nature*. 2005;434: 79–83.

Crick F, Koch C. The hidden mind. A postscript to "The problem of consciousness." *Sci Am*. 2002:272.

Hoffmann DDW. *Visual intelligence: How we create what we see*. New York: W Norton & Company; 1998.

Öhman A, Mineka S. Fears, phobias, and preparedness: Toward an evolved module of fear and fear learning. *Psychol Rev*. 2001;108(3):483–522.

Shepard RN. *Mind sights: Original visual illusions, ambiguities, and other anomalies*. New York: WH Freeman and Company; 1990.

2. What does the brain know about the body?

Boucher O, Rouleau I, Escudier F, et al. Neuropsychological performance before and after partial or complete insulectomy in patients with epilepsy. *Epilepsy Behav*. 2015;43:53–60.

Craig AD. How do you feel? Interoception: The sense of the physiological condition of the body. *Nat Rev Neurosci*. 2002;3(8):655–66.

Ehrsson HH. The experimental induction of out-of-body experiences. *Science.* 2007;317(5841):1048.

Jones CL, Ward J, Critchley HD. The neuropsychological impact of insular cortex lesions. *J Neurol Neurosurg Psychiatry.* 2010;81(6):611–18.

Petrovic P, Castellanos FX. Top-down dysregulation: From ADHD to emotional instability. *Front Behav Neurosci.* 2016;10:70.

Ramachandran VS, Blakeslee S. *Phantoms in the brain: Probing the mysteries of the human mind.* New York: William Morrow; 1998.

Sacks O. *A leg to stand on.* New York: Simon & Schuster; 1983.

Schedlowski M, Pacheco-López G. The learned immune response: Pavlov and beyond. *Brain Behav Immun.* 2010;24(2):176–85.

Van der Hoort B, Guterstam A, Ehrsson HH. Being Barbie: The size of one's own body determines the perceived size of the world. *PLoS ONE.* 2011;6(5):e20195.

3. Our inner defense systems

Chen GY, Nuñez G. Sterile inflammation: Sensing and reacting to damage. *Nat Rev Immun.* 2010;10(12):826–37.

Goldsby RA, Kindt TJ, Kuby J, Osborne BA. *Immunology.* 5th ed. New York: WH Freeman and Company; 2003.

Lekander M. Ecological immunology: The role of the immune system in psychology and neuroscience. *Eur Psychol.* 2002;7(2):98–115.

Lekander M. Stress och immunsystemet. In: Theorell T, ed. *Psykosocial miljö och stress.* Stockholm: Studentlitteratur; 2012.

Lekander M, Olgart Höglund C. Stress och allergi. *Allergi i Praxis.* 2008;3:30–6.

Trambas CM, Griffiths GM. Delivering the kiss of death. *Nat Immun.* 2003;4(5):399–403.

4. The sickness response

Beutler B, Rietschel ET. Innate immune sensing and its roots: The story of endotoxin. *Nat Rev Immun.* 2003;3(2):169–76.

Dantzer R, Kelley KW. Twenty years of research on cytokine-induced sickness behavior. *Brain Behav Immun.* 2007;21(2):153–60.

Hart BL. Biological basis of the behavior of sick animals. *Neurosci Biobehav Rev.* 1988;12(2):123–37.

Karshikoff B, Jensen KB, Kosek E, et al. Why sickness hurts: A central mechanism for pain induced by peripheral inflammation. *Brain Behav Immun.* 2016;57:38–46.

Karshikoff B, Lekander M, Soop A, et al. Modality and sex differences in pain sensitivity during human endotoxemia. *Brain Behav Immun.* 2015;46:35–43.

Karshikoff B, Sundelin T, Lasselin J. Role of inflammation in human fatigue: Relevance of multidimensional assessments and potential neuronal mechanisms. *Front Immun.* 2017;8:21.

Lasselin J, Elsenbruch S, Lekander M, et al. Mood disturbance during experimental endotoxemia: Predictors of state anxiety as a psychological component of sickness behavior. *Brain Behav Immun.* 2016;57:30–7.

Lekander M. Ecological immunology: The role of the immune system in psychology and neuroscience. *Eur Psychol.* 2002;7(2):98–115.

Selye H. *The stress of life.* Revised ed. New York: McGraw-Hill; 1976.

5. Disgust and prejudice in disease defense

Bomers MK, van Agtmael MA, Luik H, van Veen MC, Vandenbroucke-Grauls CM, Smulders YM. Using a dog's superior olfactory sensitivity to identify Clostridium difficile in stools and patients: Proof of principle study. *Br Med J.* 2012;345:e7396.

Chapman HA, Kim DA, Susskind JM, Anderson AK. In bad taste: Evidence for the oral origins of moral disgust. *Science.* 2009;323(5918):1222–6.

Faulkner J, Schaller M, Park JH, Duncan LA. Evolved disease-avoidance mechanisms and contemporary xenophobic attitudes. *Group Process Intergroup Relat.* 2004;7(4): 333–53.

Frumin I, Perl O, Endevelt-Shapira Y, et al. A social chemosignaling function for human handshaking. *eLife.* 2015;4:e05154.

Henderson AJ, Lasselin J, Lekander M, et al. Skin colour changes during experimentally-induced sickness. *Brain Behav Immun.* 2017;60:312–18.

Huang JY, Sedlovskaya A, Ackerman JM, Bargh JA. Immunizing against prejudice: Effects of disease protection on attitudes toward out-groups. *Psychol Sci.* 2011;22(12):1550–6.

Laska, M. Human olfactory capabilities in comparison to those of animals. In: Buettner A, ed. *Springer handbook of odor.* New York: Springer; 2017:667–81.

Lasselin J, Sundelin T, Wayne PM, et al. Biological motion during inflammation in humans. *Brain Behav Immun.* 2020;84:147–53.

Lippi G, Cervellin G. Canine olfactory detection of cancer versus laboratory testing: Myth or opportunity? *Clin Chem Lab Med.* 2012;50(3):435–9.

Navarrete CD, Fessler DMT, Eng SJ. Elevated ethnocentrism in the first trimester of pregnancy. *Evol Hum Behav.* 2007;28(1):60–5.

Navarrete CD, Fessler DMT. Disease avoidance and ethnocentrism: The effects of disease vulnerability and disgust sensitivity on intergroup attitudes. *Evol Hum Behav.* 2006;27(4):270–82.

Olsson A, Ebert JP, Banaji MR, Phelps EA. The role of social groups in the persistence of learned fear. *Science.* 2005;309(5735):785–7.

Olsson MJ, Lundström JN, Kimball BA, et al. The scent of disease: Human body odor contains an early chemosensory cue of sickness. *Psychol Sci.* 2014;25(3): 817–23.

Stephen ID, Law Smith MJ, Stirrat MR, Perrett DI. Facial skin coloration affects perceived health of human faces. *Folia Primatol.* 2009;30(6):845–57.

Suedfeld P, Schaller M. Authoritarianism and the Holocaust: Some cognitive and affective implications. In: Newman LS, Erber R, eds. *Understanding genocide: The social psychology of the Holocaust*. Oxford: Oxford University Press; 2002:68–90.

Sundelin T, Karshikoff B, Axelsson E, Höglund CO, Lekander M, Axelsson J. Sick man walking: Perception of health status from body motion. *Brain Behav Immun*. 2015;48:53–6.

Thornhill R, Fincher CL. *The parasite-stress theory of values and sociality. Infectious disease, history and human values worldwide*. New York: Springer; 2014.

Xu X, Zuo X, Wang X, Han S. Do you feel my pain? Racial group membership modulates empathic neural responses. *J Neurosci*. 2009;29(26):8525–9.

6. How do you rate your general health?

Andreasson A, Karshikoff B, Lidberg L, et al. The effect of a transient immune activation on subjective health perception in two placebo controlled randomised experiments. *PLoS ONE*. 2019;14(3):e0212313.

Andreasson A, Unden AL, Elofsson S, von Essen J, Nilsson L-G, Lekander M. Association between cytokines, self-perceived health, and affect in women. *Psychosom Med*. 2007;69(1):A96.

Arnberg FK, Lekander M, Morey JN, Segerstrom SC. Self-rated health and interleukin-6: Longitudinal relationships in older adults. *Brain Behav Immun*. 2016;54:226–32.

Benyamini Y. Why does self-rated health predict mortality? An update on current knowledge and a research agenda for psychologists. *Psychol Health*. 2011;26(11):1407–13.

Debruyne H, Portzky M, Van den Eynde F, Audenaert K. Cotard's syndrome: A review. *Curr Psychiatry Rep*. 2009;11(3):197–202.

Ganna A, Ingelsson E. 5-year mortality predictors in 498,103 UK Biobank participants: A prospective population-based study. *Lancet*. 2015;386(9993):533–40.

Helldén A, Odar-Cederlöf I, Larsson K, Fehrman-Ekholm I, Lindén T. Death delusion. *Br Med J*. 2007;335:1305.

Jylhä M, Guralnik J, Ferrucci L, Jokela J, Heikkinen E. Is self-rated health comparable across cultures and genders? *J Gerontol: Soc Sci*. 1998;53B:S144–52.

Lekander M, Andreasson AN, Kecklund G, et al. Subjective health perception in healthy young men changes in response to experimentally restricted sleep and subsequent recovery sleep. *Brain Behav Immun*. 2013;34:43–6.

Lekander M, Elofsson S, Neve IM, Hansson LO, Undén AL. Self-rated health is related to levels of circulating cytokines. *Psychosom Med*. 2004;66(4):559–63.

Organization for Economic Cooperation and Development (OECD). Health at a glance 2019: OECD indicators. https://www.oecd-ilibrary.org/sites/4dd50c09-en/1/1/1/index.html?itemId=/content/publication/4dd50c09-en&mimeType=text/html&_csp_=82587932df7c06a6a3f9dab95304095d&itemIGO=oecd&itemContentType=book. Accessed August 30, 2020.

Petrovic P. *Känslostormar: Emotionell instabilitet och hjärnan*. Stockholm: Natur & Kultur; 2015.

Petrovic P, Castellanos FX. Top-down dysregulation—From ADHD to emotional instability. *Front Behav Neurosci.* 2016;10:70.

Petrovic P, Ekman CJ, Klahr J, et al. Significant grey matter changes in a region of the orbitofrontal cortex in healthy participants predicts emotional dysregulation. *Soc Cogn Affect Neurosci.* 2016;11(7):1041–9.

Ruthig JC, Chipperfield JG, Payne BJ. A five-year study of older adults' health incongruence: Consistency, functional changes and subsequent survival. *Psychol Health.* 2011;26(11):1463–78.

Schnittker J, Bacak V. The increasing predictive validity of self-rated health. *PLoS ONE.* 2014;9(1):e84933.

Schulze L, Domes G, Krüger A, et al. Neuronal correlates of cognitive reappraisal in borderline patients with affective instability. *Biol Psychiatry.* 2011;69(6):564–73.

Simpson JR, Ongür D, Akbudak E, et al. The emotional modulation of cognitive processing: An fMRI study. *J Cogn Neurosci.* 2000;12(Suppl 2):157–70.

Singh-Manoux A, Martikainen P, Ferrie J, Zins M, Marmot M, Goldberg M. What does self-rated health measure? Results from the British Whitehall II and French Gazel cohort studies. *J Epidemiol Community Health.* 2006;60(4):364–72.

Undén A-L, Elofsson S. Health from the patient's point of view. How does it relate to the physician's judgement? *Fam Pract.* 2001;18:174–80.

7. Feeling sick and other emotions

Axelsson J, Sundelin T, Olsson MJ, Sorjonen K, Axelsson C, Lasselin J, Lekander M. Identification of acutely sick people and facial cues of sickness. Proceedings of the Royal Society B: Biological Sciences. 2018;285(1870).

Ekman P. Moods, emotions and traits. In: Ekman P, Davidson RJ, eds. *The nature of emotions.* Oxford: Oxford University Press; 1994:56–8.

Frijda, N. *The emotions.* Cambridge: Cambridge University Press; 1986.

LeDoux J. Rethinking the emotional brain. *Neuron.* 2012;73(4):653–76.

Modinos G, Ormel J, Aleman A. Activation of anterior insula during self-reflection. *PLoS ONE.* 2009;4(2):e4618.

Öhman A, Mineka S. Fears, phobias, and preparedness: toward an evolved module of fear and fear learning. *Psychol Rev.* 2001;108(3):483–522.

Sarolidou G, Axelsson J, Sundelin T, et al. Emotional expressions of the sick face. *Brain Behav Immun.* 2019;80:286–91.

8. Can you affect your perceived health?

Adler A, Seligman MEP. Using wellbeing for public policy: Theory, measurement, and recommendations. *Int J Well.* 2016;6(1):1–35.

Andreasson A, Schiller H, Akerstedt T, Berntson E, Kecklund G, Lekander M. Brief report: Contemplate your symptoms and re-evaluate your health. A study on working adults. *J Health Psychol.* Sep;24(11):1562–7.

Asmundson GJG, Taylor S. *It's not all in your head: How worrying about your health could be making you sick and what you can do about it.* New York: Guilford; 2005.

Craig AD. The sentient self. *Brain Struct Funct.* 2010;214(5–6):563–77.

Crum AJ, Langer EJ. Mind-set matters: Exercise and the placebo effect. *Psychol Sci.* 2007;18(2):165–71.

Hayman JA. Darwin's illness revisited. *Br Med J.* 2009;339:b4968.

Hedman E, Andersson G, Andersson E, et al. Internet-based cognitive-behavioural therapy for severe health anxiety: Randomised controlled trial. *Br J Psychiatry.* 2011;198:230–6.

Hedman E, Lekander M, Karshikoff B, Ljótsson B, Axelsson E, Axelsson J. Health anxiety in a disease-avoidance framework: Investigation of anxiety, disgust and disease perception in response to sickness cues. *J Abnorm Psychol.* 2016;125(7):868–78.

Hedman-Lagerlof E, Axelsson E, Andersson E, Ljotsson B, Andreasson A, Lekander M. The impact of exposure-based cognitive behavior therapy for severe health anxiety on self-rated health: Results from a randomized trial. *J Psychosom Res.* 2017;103:9–14.

Helweg HHC. *H.C. Andersen: En psykiatrisk studie,* 2nd ed. Köpenhamn: H Hagerups Forlag; 1954.

Jensen KB, Srinivasan P, Spaeth R, et al. Overlapping structural and functional brain changes in patients with long-term exposure to fibromyalgia pain. *Arthritis Rheumatol.* 2013;65(12):3293–303.

Kahneman D. *Thinking, fast and slow.* New York: Farrar, Straus and Giroux; 2011.

Kringelbach ML. The human orbitofrontal cortex: Linking reward to hedonic experience. *Nat Rev Neurosci.* 2005;6(9):691–702.

Lindsäter E, Axelsson E, Salomonsson S, et al. Internet-based cognitive behavioral therapy for chronic stress: A randomized controlled trial. *Psychother Psychosom.* 2018;87(5):296–305.

Olatunji BO. Selective effects of excessive engagement in health-related behaviours on disgust propensity. *Cogn Emot.* 2015;29(5):882–99.

Schoenberg PL, David AS. Biofeedback for psychiatric disorders: A systematic review. *Appl Psychophysiol Biofeedback.* 2014;39:109–35.

University of Cambridge. Darwin Correspondence Project. October 16, 2016. https://www.darwinproject.ac.uk

Uylings HB, Sanz-Arigita EJ, de Vos K, Pool CW, Evers P, Rajkowska G. 3-D cyto-architectonic parcellation of human orbitofrontal cortex correlation with post-mortem MRI. *Psychiatry Res.* 2010;183(1):1–20.

9. How society affects our health

Atun R. Transitioning health systems for multimorbidity. *Lancet.* 2015;386(9995):721–2.

Atun R, Jaffar S, Nishtar S, et al. Improving responsiveness of health systems to non-communicable diseases. *Lancet.* 2013;381(9867):690–7.

Basch E, Torda P, Adams K. Standards for patient-reported outcome-based performance measures. *J Am Med Assoc.* 2013;310(2):139–40.

Brundage M, Blazeby J, Revicki D, et al. Patient-reported outcomes in randomized clinical trials: Development of ISOQOL reporting standards. *Qual Life Res.* 2013;22(6):1161–75.

Clark DM. Realizing the mass public benefit of evidence-based psychological therapies: The IAPT Program. *Ann Rev Clin Psychol.* 2018;14:159–83.

Ernst E. How much of CAM is based on research evidence? *Evid Based Complement Alternat Med.* 2011;2011(501):676490.

Ernst E, Pittler M, Wider B. *The desktop guide to complementary and alternative medicine.* 2nd ed. Elsevier; 2006.

Global Burden of Disease Study 2013 Collaborators. Global, regional, and national incidence, prevalence, and years lived with disability for 301 acute and chronic diseases and injuries in 188 countries, 1990–2013: A systematic analysis for the Global Burden of Disease Study 2013. *Lancet.* 2015;386(9995):743–800.

Global Burden of Disease Study 2017 Collaborators. Global, regional, and national incidence, prevalence, and years lived with disability for 354 diseases and injuries for 195 countries and territories, 1990–2017: A systematic analysis for the Global Burden of Disease Study 2017. *Lancet.* 2018;392(10159):1789–858.

Hont G. Kultursjukdomar irriterar och utmanar läkarkåren. Intervju med Karin Johannisson. *Läkartidningen.* 2007;46:3432–4.

Johannisson K. *Melankoliska rum: Om ångest, leda och sårbarhet i förfluten tid och nutid.* Falun: Albert Bonniers Förlag; 2009.

Layard R, Clark DM. *Thrive: The power of evidence-based psychological therapies.* London: Allen Lane; 2014.

Mann T. *The magic mountain.* London: Secker & Warburg; 1924.

National Quality Forum. Patient reported outcomes (PROs) in performance measurement. 2013.

PROMIS. Health measures: Introduction to PROMIS. August 16, 2020. http://www.healthmeasures.net/explore-measurement-systems/promis/intro-to-promis

Sachs L. *Onda ögat eller bakterier—turkiska invandrarkvinnors möte med svensk sjukvård.* Stockholm: Liber; 1983.

Schweder RA, LeVine RA. *Culture theory: Essays on mind, self and emotion.* Cambridge: Cambridge University Press; 1984.

Tricco AC, Ivers NM, Grimshaw JM, et al. Effectiveness of quality improvement strategies on the management of diabetes: A systematic review and meta-analysis. *Lancet.* 2012;379(9833):2252–61.

Tybur JM, Inbar Y, Aarøe L, et al. Parasite stress and pathogen avoidance relate to distinct dimensions of political ideology across 30 nations. *Proc Natl Acad Sci.* 2016;113(44):12408–13.

Van Tilburg MA, Becht MC, Vingerhoets AJ. Self-reported crying during the menstrual cycle: Sign of discomfort and emotional turmoil or erroneous beliefs? *J Psychosom Obstet Gynecol.* 2003;24(4):247–55.

World Health Organization. People-centered health care. A policy framework. 2007.

World Health Organization. Global burden of mental disorders and the need for a comprehensive, coordinated response from health and social sectors at the country level. 1 December 2011.

10. Perhaps it's not that bad?

Asmundson GJG, Taylor S. *It's not all in your head: How worrying about your health could be making you sick and what you can do about it.* New York: Guilford; 2005.

Crum AJ, Leibowitz KA, Verghese A. Making mindset matter. *Br Med J.* 2017;356:j674.

Hedman E, Linde J, Leiler P, Andersson E, Axelsson E, Ljótsson B. *Tänk om jag är sjuk!* Stockholm: Natur & Kultur; 2016.

Merckelbach H, Jelicic M, Pieters M. Misinformation increases symptom reporting: A test-retest study. *JRSM Short Rep.* 2011;2(10):75.

Index

Figures are indicated by *f* following the page number. Notes are denoted by the letter 'n' and note number following the page number.